MULTIFAITH CARE FOR SICK AND DYING CHILDREN AND THEIR FAMILIES

of related interest

Exploring Spiritual Care with Sick Children and Young People
Paul Nash, Sally Nash, Kathryn Darby with Rebecca Nye
ISBN 978 1 84905 389 1
eISBN 978 1 78450 063 4

Spiritual Care in Practice
Case Studies in Healthcare Chaplaincy
Edited by George Fitchett and Steve Nolan
Foreword by Christina M. Puchalski
ISBN 978 1 84905 976 3
eISBN 978 0 85700 876 3

Making Sense of Spirituality in Nursing and Health Care Practice
An Interactive Approach
2nd edition
Wilfred McSherry
Foreword by Keith Cash
ISBN 978 1 84310 365 3
eISBN 978 1 84642 530 1

Spirituality in Health Care Contexts
Edited by Helen Orchard
ISBN 978 1 85302 969 1
eISBN 978 0 85700 177 1

The Spirit of the Child
Revised Edition
David Hay
With Rebecca Nye
ISBN 978 1 84310 371 4
eISBN 978 1 84642 473 1

MULTIFAITH CARE FOR SICK AND DYING CHILDREN AND THEIR FAMILIES

A MULTIDISCIPLINARY GUIDE

Written and Edited by Paul Nash, Madeleine Parkes and Zamir Hussain

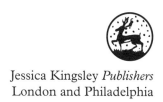

Jessica Kingsley *Publishers*
London and Philadelphia

Box on page 76 is reproduced with kind permission from Hinduism Today.
Box on page 100 is reproduced from an interview in *The Texas Jewish Post* with kind permission from Rabbi Lord Jonathan Sacks.
Box on page 110 is reproduced from an article by Rabbi Aron Moss with kind permission from Chabad.org.

First published in 2015
by Jessica Kingsley Publishers
73 Collier Street
London N1 9BE, UK
and
400 Market Street, Suite 400
Philadelphia, PA 19106, USA

www.jkp.com

PLYMOUTH UNIVERSITY

9 009686060

Library of Congress Cataloging in Publication Data
Nash, Paul, 1959- , author.
  Multifaith care for sick and dying children and their families : a multi-disciplinary guide / Paul Nash,
Madeleine Parkes, and Zamir Hussain.
     p. cm.
  Includes bibliographical references and index.
  ISBN 978-1-84905-606-9 (alk. paper)
  1. Medical care--Religious aspects. 2. Child health services--Great Britain. I. Parkes, Madeleine, author.
II. Hussain, Zamir, author. III. Title.
  [DNLM: 1. Culturally Competent Care--Great Britain. 2. Religion and Medicine--Great Britain. 3.
Adolescent--Great Britain. 4. Child--Great Britain. 5. Infant--Great Britain. 6. Pastoral Care--Great
Britain. 7. Professional-Patient Relations--Great Britain. BL 65.M4]
  BL65.M4N37 2015
  362.19892--dc23
                         2014047758

British Library Cataloguing in Publication Data
A CIP catalogue record for this book is available from the British Library

ISBN 978 1 84905 606 9
eISBN 978 1 78450 072 6

Printed and bound in Great Britain

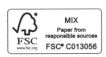

*To the children, young people and staff of Birmingham
Children's Hospital, and at hospitals and hospices around
the world, whose stories are represented in this book*

CONTENTS

ACKNOWLEDGEMENTS

Thanks to the Paediatric Chaplaincy Network of Great Britain and Ireland for their support in developing this book, and for all who shared stories and insights to make it possible in this network and beyond.

Thank you to the Multifaith Healthcare Group for the contributions of their representatives.

Thanks to Sara Reynolds and Rachel Hill-Brown for their ideas for faith-based celebrations, which have all been used in hospital contexts.

Thanks to the Society for Promoting Christian Knowledge (SPCK) and Wild Goose Worship Group for permission to use material in Chapter 8.

Thanks to Sally Nash who did the final compilation and editing of the book and supported Paul from the initial idea and visit to Jessica Kingsley to completion.

We are grateful for the support of Birmingham Children's Hospital in establishing Red Balloon Resources, which publishes a range of books, booklets and cards to support multifaith religious care of children, young people and their families. Red Balloon Resources can be contacted at rbr@bch.nhs.uk.

INTRODUCTION

Paul Nash

This book seeks to address issues of care in our increasingly multifaith cultural context. It is written with awareness that being sensitive and attentive to the religious and spiritual needs of a child and family are intrinsic to holistic care[1] and that in the English context is a National Health Service (NHS) directive.[2, 3] While there are some very helpful books and hospital websites explaining how those of different faiths may wish to be cared for when in hospital, most of this material focuses on adults. Our experience at Birmingham Children's Hospital (BCH) is that some of this information is inaccurate with regard to babies, children and young people and sometimes potentially upsetting to families if applied.

It is hoped that this book will be helpful to healthcare professionals, including chaplains and others working with babies, children, young people and their families in hospitals, hospices and the community. We seek to look at different aspects of care including day-to-day, palliative, end-of-life and bereavement care.

Why have we written this book?

Almost all the information and training packs on multifaith healthcare have been written with caring for adults in mind. And, although much of the information is the same for adults and children, there are major important differences within each of the world religions covered in this book; for example, adult Hindus are always cremated, but babies can be buried. We have also sought, for probably the first time in this kind of book, to explore the interactions between religious belief, child development and illness in healthcare settings, and the implications of these interactions.

In wanting to offer appropriate, respectful care to patients and their families who have a faith that is different from ours, we may have adopted one of the three classic responses to difficult situations: fight, flight or freeze. If we enable staff to feel confident and equipped to care for those who are different from themselves in areas where faith is pertinent then this should minimize these sorts of responses to what can be challenging circumstances such as a dying child. With the growing cultures of respect, compassion, risk assessment, and complaint and compensation, it is to the benefit and interest of every caring institution, organization and service to take the objectives and content of this book seriously.

The serious illness or death of a child is probably one of the most traumatic or devastating things that a parent can experience. Their grief and sorrow may be exacerbated if their faith is not taken seriously and actions are taken, usually unknowingly, by staff which contradict their beliefs and religious practices. It is beyond the scope of this book to discuss the way that pastoral and spiritual care may be helpful but the hope is that through understanding how faith impacts sickness and dying children, young people and families will receive more appropriate care.

In researching paediatric religious and spiritual care, we found that some of the distinctiveness was around more support with families; care of children in the spectrum of their development levels; working as a part of multidisciplinary teams; supporting staff; a robust understanding of suffering. Some of these issues and themes we seek to address in this book.

As precise as we have sought to be in this book, we are not imagining we are covering the spectrum of all the different traditions within each of these world faiths. We hope to make a contribution to taking children and young people as patients of faith seriously, and not just treating them like 'little adults'. There is very little published in this area and what we are offering are some reflections on the topic, exploring some hypotheses which need to be tested as part of a bigger project and ongoing dialogue. We have invited others from the UK and beyond to contribute illustrations to the book.

Our context: Birmingham Children's Hospital NHS Foundation Trust

BCH has 365 beds, 3500 staff and is located in the centre of Great Britain's second largest city. The population of Birmingham in 2011, the date of the last census, was 1.07 million with a higher than national average, 22.8 per cent, of 0–15-year-olds. Of the residents, 46.1 per cent identified themselves as Christian, 21.8 per cent as Muslim, 19.3 per cent said they had no religion, 3 per cent as Sikh, 2.1 per cent as Hindu, 0.4 per cent as Buddhist and 0.2 per cent as Jewish.

Definitions

It may be helpful at the beginning of the book to distinguish between different types of care:

- *Religious care* relates specifically to the tenets, practices, rituals and conventions of a particular religious faith.

- *Spiritual care* involves facilitating an individual's engagement with the existential questions of life, which involve identity, purpose and the potentiality of a relationship with or connectedness to a transcendent dimension or a sense of the sacred.

- *Pastoral care* is a term used beyond a Christian context, for example in schools, and refers to care given to address the cares, concerns, problems, needs and issues of an individual or family.

- *Cultural care* may or may not be connected to religious faith but can have an impact on practice, and people of the same faith but from different cultures may express their faith differently, for example in colour of clothing for funerals. There may also be cultural shock to contend with if patients and their families become ill when travelling; the location of our institutions may determine the extent to which this is a problem.

However, it needs to be noted that within the NHS in the UK spiritual care is used as a term which may be perceived as including all these dimensions.[4] This can also be true in the USA and other places around the world.

I hope it goes without saying that we are not assuming all children to have a religious belief, and, even those in families where religious belief is held in high regard, that the children and young people follow these beliefs in the same way as their families or even at all.

When we use the term 'healthcare', we seek to include hospital, community and hospice care, and when we use the term 'children', we mean the full age spectrum of the patients in a children's hospital.

Overview of the book

The first chapter offers a set of objectives and values for multifaith care; they are derived from Paul's work in chaplaincy in multicultural contexts over the years. They are a work in progress as experience, further study and reflection mean that they evolve over time. Chapters 2–7 cover six major world faiths; they are presented in alphabetical order and include what is distinctive in paediatric care and ideas on how that faith may be celebrated with children and young people in a hospital or similar context.[5] Chapter 8, using a case study of one family's experience, explores spiritual care and how this may be different to religious care, sometimes complementary and sometimes stand-alone. Chapter 9 is a Buddhist mother's reflection on her experiences in hospital and her reflections on the religious care she received. Chapter 10 seeks to draw together a way forward to integrate religious belief and healthcare, and the Conclusion offers some summary principles.

Notes

1   Department of Health (2010) *Equity and Excellence: Liberating the NHS* (White Paper). Norwich: TSO. Available at www.gov.uk/government/publications/liberating-the-nhs-white-paper, accessed on 17 February 2014.

2   National Institute for Health and Clinical Excellence (2005) *Guidance on Cancer Services: Improving Outcomes in Children and Young People with Cancer.* London: NHS. Available at http://guidance.nice.org.uk/CSGCYP/Guidance/pdf/English, accessed on 8 February 2013.

3   SYWDU (2003) *Caring for the Spirit.* South Yorkshire Workforce Development Confederation. Available at www.nhs-chaplaincy-spiritualcare.org.uk/Caringforthe%20Spirit2003.pdf, accessed on 17 February 2014.

4   Cobb, M. (2005) *The Hospital Chaplain's Handbook.* Norwich: Canterbury Press.

5   In the UK, Baker Ross (www.bakerross.co.uk) have lots of faith-specific resources to celebrate festivals. Interfaith Calendar (www.interfaithcalendar.org/index.htm) has a list of festivals.

1

FIVE KEY VALUES AND OBJECTIVES FOR MULTIFAITH CARE

Paul Nash

I have been a paediatric chaplain since 2002. Before this I spent five years working in a church in inner-city Birmingham as a Christian priest and before that in youth work for 15 years. Chaplaincy was not as straightforward as working in a church, and at first I found this difficult to handle. Being of one faith was hard enough, but the mixture of faiths I encountered in the hospital sometimes made it confusing to know where to start. Within the chaplaincy team we have done a Buddhist–Christian end-of-life blessing for a teenager and our Roman Catholic chaplain took a Sikh funeral. We have learnt that what is appropriate and sometimes expected is to remain true to our own tradition while being sensitive to others' perspectives. This chapter represents my own approach to multifaith care. It is the product of my experience and reflections of working with other healthcare professionals, and it reflects the culture that I have sought to develop within BCH and our chaplaincy team. It is offered as one way of understanding multifaith care and as a starting point or example for developing your own principles and practice.

Our model: the starfish story

As the old man walked along the beach, he noticed a young woman ahead of him picking up starfish and flinging them into the sea. Finally catching up with the young woman, he asked her why she was doing this. The answer was that the stranded starfish would die if left until the morning. 'But the beach goes on for miles and there are millions of starfish' countered the other. 'How can you make any difference?' The young woman looked at the starfish in her hand and threw it safely in the waves. 'It will make a difference to this one,' she said.[1]

This story gives a good indication of the purpose, values and attitude towards our work. We seek to make a difference to patients (children, young people), families, staff and the wider community. What is important is to make a correct diagnosis of needs and offer the appropriate care which, as we explained in the Introduction, may be religious, spiritual, pastoral or cultural alongside the medical.

Explanation and application of the starfish metaphor

The arms of the starfish represent core principles and values. This is symbolized by the upper side of the starfish, what you see when the starfish is on the beach. Like a starfish, there is also an underside to our work: that which you cannot see but know is there because that is how the starfish moves, holds on and feeds.

The five arms of the starfish will each be represented by a principle. The making a difference is expressed in how we apply these principles. The underbelly represents our values, why we do what we do, what we believe. It shapes our practice and our principles. It helps us move and helps us hold on to our ground. It is often unseen but profoundly affects our practice. Each of the five principles and underbelly are discussed below:

Principle	Underbelly
1. Creative, focused competence	Secure vocational identity
2. Global, inclusive connectivity	Comfortable on the margins
3. Courageously challenging	Vulnerable availability
4. Sustaining, accessible compassion	Self-care
5. Celebrating and championing diversity	Understanding and appreciating uniqueness

1. Creative, focused competence

Be informed: religious and cultural literacy

To care appropriately we need to know the relevant information. Within a hospital context we know what religion families wish to record themselves as. This enables us to take faith into account in planning care. What we may need to do is to develop our cultural and religious literacy to offer the best possible care. This involves such things as:

- how respect is shown

- greetings, physical contact, privacy

- status, deference in family dynamics

- attitude towards health, illness, suffering and death

- dress

- food, diet

- prayer needs

- core beliefs and values

- potential clashes

- community leadership and authority structures

- how to identify someone's faith or cultural background

- demographics.

Much of this will be covered in subsequent faith chapters. Please also see Appendix 1 for a crib sheet that summarizes all the key issues.

Understanding how care can compound or diminish religious distress is an essential skill and knowledge for all healthcare staff. Why and how it is important to some faiths that same-gender care is usually appropriate for their child once they have reached puberty will save staff from a risk of offending and lessen stress in patients and families. Religious coping and even thriving can be our goal in our healthcare.

Aim to become effective in focused holistic care

We have a growing multifaith population in many of our hospitals and hospices and if our institutions are going to fulfil their responsibilities, the make-up of the chaplaincy team should reflect this.

Multidisciplinary care staff can have competency in paediatric religious care but, in addition, it is our experience that when there are difficult situations, many patients and families prefer to receive religious care from chaplains of their own faith tradition. We appreciate the financial considerations, but when put against the potential risks of the offence and negligence of religious needs not being taken into account, as well as the enhanced sense of peace patients and families will feel that their needs are understood and accommodated, it is money well spent.

We have also sought to equip multidisciplinary staff in religious and spiritual care and have engaged in some research on the spiritual and religious needs of young people to help provide an evidence base for this. What emerged from this included:

- raising awareness of what is involved in spiritual care and ways to facilitate this

- finding new and creative ways of assessing spiritual and religious needs which are relevant for children and young people would be helpful, and assessment needs to be ongoing

- often trying to assess need involves an intervention too

- promoting wellbeing and connectedness through things like gestures of kindness, taking time to listen, normalizing activities (doing things which other young people do)

- where it is possible offer choices which help give patients a sense of control

- positive culture setting and building community

- facilitating, where possible, opportunities to give back

- help young people to explore their worldview

- as far as possible enhancing the quality of the physical environment as this contributes to wellbeing.[2, 3]

It is also important that we realize we know in part but will never know everything and that we are willing to admit our limitations and refer on when necessary. How comfortable a staff member may be in discussing religious and spiritual issues may determine their skill in offering religious care.

Celebrating and using what we have in common

During several multifaith projects, we have had cause to discuss what we have in common. One of the best examples of this was when we worked with The Kings Fund on a bereavement project called 'Enhancing the Healing Environment'. The objective was to improve the environment for bereaved parents. This included making serious changes and modifications to our bereavement viewing suite, The Rainbow Room, which involved incorporating a small garden area into the space. To add beauty, comfort and inspiration to this area it was decide to have a wood carving placed onto the garden wall. Our Multi Faith and Cultural Advisory Group (MF&CAG) met to see if we could find and agree an image that would be appreciated by most major faiths. We had a rigorous discussion and many images such as faces (not acceptable to Muslims) were dismissed. I shared the idea of the whirlpool of grief as an image many bereaved families identified with, and we quickly discovered that water, especially running, moving water, was not offensive to anyone around the table, but actually had a positive connotation and healing qualities in many faiths. So this is what we commissioned, and it is still appreciated today.[4]

In subsequent discussions around our multifaith Celebrate project and events,[5] light is a positive image in many world religions. The golden rule 'do to others as you would like to be done to you' is also one of the most well-known commonalities.

Our hospital has always been committed to high quality bereavement care. We have also sought to do well, where some aspects of the hospital frequently find it difficult, in knowing how to deal with faith-specific bereavement care. One of the main reasons this may be so is that the death of a child is tragic and staff come to work to save and give life. In the light of this and as a reflection that religious leaders have something unique to offer around confidence in death, we have developed a religious bereavement care pathway that is comprehensive and respectful to multifaith bereavement care of our families and the pastoral support and training needs of our staff.[6]

Underbelly: Secure vocational identity

I am entitled to be true to my beliefs and values…and so are other staff.

When I became a chaplain I spent some time thinking through how my beliefs and values as a healthcare professional worked out in this new setting. These are some of the lessons and insights I have found important in being true to my own tradition:

- Have an attitude of humility towards self and tradition.

- Be open to learn from others and draw on their tradition.

- Be honest with yourself and articulate the tensions.

- Learn to live with the differences.

- Offer the same generosity to others that you would like for yourself.

- Find a way to express your beliefs and values while following principles of respect and non-oppression.

- Value diversity.

- Understand and honour your roots.

- Be prepared to be what's needed.

- Be aware your tradition moves and/or you may revisit or reinvent tradition.

- Realize you might change or need to change.

- Negotiate risk.

- Be the virtuous leader your tradition would encourage.

Motives

This has been an essential area for me to reflect on. Where might I have any temptation to transfer and project my values and baggage onto other? Why am I doing what I am doing? I have sought to do this with honesty and not just give the seemingly correct answer or process. Self-awareness is an essential skill to have within multifaith healthcare. I have learnt that I need to be honest with my inner life regardless of what I find; denial is not a useful attribute in this or any type of leadership. We have no right to push or deny the religious rights or care of our patients and perhaps need to ask ourselves, 'Do I have areas of bias – positive and negative?' or 'Do I have a tendency to over-promote?' Vocational identity is an area which may be helpfully explored in non-clinical supervision or through a mentoring relationship.

2. Global, inclusive connectivity

Integration not marginalization

Applying this principle to a patient's religious care is essential to their holistic wellbeing and is found in one expression or another in almost all healthcare professionals' standards. Sometimes the religious and everyday aspects of their lives intertwine, for example with dietary regulations and the content of medicine. If religious needs are marginalized then this can be experienced as a lack of respect. However, careful attention needs to be given to ensure that staff are equipped to offer such care. Austin writes, 'A lack of collaboration among healthcare professionals has been complicated by a lack of understanding about professional functions and basic concepts of spirituality in healthcare treatment.'[7] Multidisciplinary care should mean that all aspects of an individual's needs are taken seriously and that no one element is marginalized. For some people their religious faith is a particular source of support for them in palliative care or in supporting family members who are sick. Ensuring that such care is integrated rather than marginalized can only be beneficial for patients. Those staff offering religious and spiritual care need to be confident about the significance of their role and may sometimes even have to advocate for patients' rights to receive such care. We explore the practice of religious assessment and whose role and responsibilities these are in Chapter 10.

Multifaith and Cultural Advisory Group

Because of the complexity of issues that can arise in relation to faith and a need for a place where such issues can be referred, BCH established a group responsible for this area, and chaplaincy facilitates the group. The responsibilities of the group include organizing multifaith and cultural celebrations throughout the hospital (examples of these are included in the relevant chapters and Appendix 2); offering advice and training on how to work with the diverse client group our hospital attracts; and taking referrals from staff on cultural and religious problems. One case we dealt with was why a Muslim young person seemed reluctant to draw in a psychology session, which was around the belief that some Muslims have that you do not draw people. I have involved my multifaith chaplaincy team in this group and other departments and individuals within the hospital. This group has now brought a much wider benefit to the hospital, as it fulfils many diversity objectives that the hospital is audited on. The terms of reference for this group can be found on the chaplaincy pages of the BCH website.

Underbelly: Comfortable on the margins

Religious care is not why children and young people are in hospital; they have come for medical care. Thus while religious care may be important to many families, those of us offering such care may be regarded by them or other staff as peripheral to the real purpose of the visit. We do well to be reminded of this and learn to be secure in this place.

3. Courageously challenging

I have realized that being challenging happens for several reasons. It can be purposeful and inadvertent.

Each of us undertakes a personal journey in relation to spirituality and religion, both personally and professionally. When I train in this area I ask these questions:

- Where have we come from?
- Where are we now?
- Where do we want to go?

My personal journey as someone who grew up in a completely white area was this:

from ignorance to...

prejudice to...

tolerance to...

acceptance to...

appreciation to...

respect, which has led me to a position of being able to offer...

effective holistic spiritual and religious healthcare.

When to challenge religious care?

The easy answer is, when we believe it is not in the best interests of the patient; it is causing them or others harm. We believe it is necessary to question aspects of religious care if we feel this is happening. This will be easier to do if we have tested ourselves on the personal journey scale above, so as to ensure we are not working out of our own prejudice. Institutionally this happens sometimes where particular families have religious beliefs, the consequence of which may be the death of the child, and in those situations the hospital may well go to court to get a ruling regarding the best interests of the patient. Our team have been involved in discussing with families such situations. An interesting case exploring some of the ethical dilemmas involved in this was that of the Maltese conjoined twins known as Jodie and Mary where the parents wanted to allow nature to take its course and thus God to decide, whereas the courts decided to separate them.[8] Male circumcision for non-medical reasons is an issue for some staff. Your institution's clinical ethics and or multifaith advisory group would be a conducive environment for these kinds of issues to be discussed.

Respect

Respect can be difficult when you disagree with someone, and this can happen within one faith as well as between faiths. We have staff and faith leaders disagree over which image best represents their religion. We may have to 'fudge' and agree to disagree, but what happens if this occurs in our hospital? Sewell notes that 'Talking about racial and cultural discrimination is often charged with fear, anger, shame, denial and avoidance. Practitioners are often reluctant to deal with these.'[9] Questions I ask myself in this regard include: Are there any ways I see my own faith as first amongst equals? Am I aware of my own bias? What does it mean to respect someone I disagree with?

Assessment of religious and spiritual needs is the responsibility of all, not just the specialists

It is acknowledged within healthcare that 'Like physical needs, spiritual needs must be assessed and responded to to promote patient wellness and comfort.'[10] When someone is first referred to a hospital or hospice there will be an assessment of their needs. Part of this assessment should involve spiritual and religious needs. This can be done by anyone and is not just the responsibility of the chaplain or other specialist. In talking about spiritual and religious needs it also gives those with no faith the opportunity to make it clear that they do not want religious care. Because faith offers resources to individuals and their families it is helpful to be aware of it and to determine hopes and expectations as they may be having an impact. It is also the responsibility of the patient to make known their religious and spiritual needs but sometimes a direct question will elicit a response when someone may not have raised it of their own accord. It is important to acknowledge that those who do not identify as religious may well have spiritual needs. This is covered in more detail in Chapter 10.

Be cautiously creative

At BCH we try to find creative ways to help people engage with spiritual and religious concerns. We have not experienced the so-called British reserve. For example, when we lead blessings or baptisms we try to make them as participative as possible, including anyone who wants to in doing something specific to mark the occasion. We have also developed some family activities to help them explore together some of their religious or spiritual needs.

Name the elephants in the room

We have found a way of creatively doing this with patients and it has been one of the most innovative projects we have done in the hospital. In partnership with the youth work department, we explored the concept of the elephant in the room through decorating decoupage elephants with their own shoebox room. This facilitated discussion of a range of significant topics around what is not being talked about in patients' care. Sometimes what needs to be raised are particularly difficult issues that may have a cultural or religious root.

Underbelly: Vulnerable availability

I am a friend of the Northumbria Community (www.northumbria community.org) and resonate with their values of intentional availability and vulnerability. When we choose to be able to challenge courageously, we put ourselves in a place of vulnerability. When we challenge prejudices and practices, we put ourselves out there. It is not a pleasant place to be. When I tell my story, I am putting myself in a position of being misunderstood; it is a risk to explain that you understand yourself to be prejudiced when your job is promoting equality and diversity. It is a risk I am willing to take as it gives others permission to explore their own journey. I have lost count of the number of staff who have thanked me for saying in bereavement teaching that frequently the most I have for our families is 'I am so sorry for your loss.' It has helped others see that their fear of not knowing what to say or not having enough to say is a common one.

Passionate but ignorant project manager

Another way I exercise vulnerable availability is to initiate projects which I know very little about. We have plans to develop resources for children, young people, families and staff. I have a good idea of why I want us to have something, when we discuss, for instance, an Islamic health and bereavement care training pack or a booklet for bereaved Sikh parents, but I am not the best placed person to say what exact words, art work, etc. should be in these resources. So I delegate to specific faith staff and play to their strengths and interests. I have chaired several faith consultations with leaders from around the country to write these resources and it is sometimes difficult to assess who is right in a disagreement. Vulnerable leadership is not inappropriate; it models credibility and shows we understand some elements but not all.

Fudge as principle

This is not my normal default as a person or as a leader. This term emerged in a conversation when researching this book. I went to interview someone who leads a Christian–Muslim youth project. We were discussing the pros and cons of explicit policies and if sometimes in this area we try to be too policy and guideline led. For instance, do we give extra holidays to celebrate religious festivals or lots of wider community funerals? A policy could be too restrictive but taking situations case by case can be seen as too arbitrary. There is merit in leaving situations like these open-ended as long as we can be fair to all the team. Our HR departments will have policies on many issues, but some are still being worked out – for example, prayers in work time.

4. Sustaining, accessible compassion

Sustaining, accessible compassion is firstly attitudinal, then worked out in practice. In the context of a children's hospital, it is an essential attitude to have in offering religious, spiritual and pastoral care for children, young people, their families and the staff. Adair quotes a Zulu proverb which says, 'I cannot hear what you say, because what you are is shouting at me.'[11] It is difficult to demonstrate compassion if dimensions of our identity get in the way. In my experience, an effective practitioner of multifaith care as well as being compassionate is honest, self-aware, trusting, respectful, gracious, vulnerable, transparent and has integrity.

I am that 'other faith'

One of the things I need to realize is that to some I am the 'other faith'. It was sobering to come out of a majority context into a place where my faith is only one of six represented in the staff team, and even less than that in the religious affiliations of the young people and children in the hospital; this brings a humbling, different perspective. When I chair the Trust's Multifaith and Cultural Advisory Group, I may represent the largest percentage of patients, but I am only one of many voices with a view on the religious care of our children, young people, families and staff. If I were to think of everyone else as 'other' and myself as the 'norm' this would reveal an awful lot about my worldview. I endeavour not to do this.

Underbelly: Self-care

If a staff member is to have sustaining, accessible compassion, self-care is an essential component. It is also a bit of an anomaly because some of the principles of looking after ourselves are contradictions in terms, as some of my care is intentionally done by other people. I am happy with self-care as a term because it puts the responsibility on me to get it organized. I have realized it is crucial to nurture my own religious and spiritual sense of wellbeing. In a previous career as a chef, the mantra that was used was 'happy chefs make happy food'. I have long believed this to be a truism and see looking after myself as a personal responsibility with corporate consequences. If I am happy in my own skin, I would suggest I am better placed to care for others. I have also found it to be important that staff are allowed to express their self-care within their faith, and not to have one size fits all. Different faiths have different models of spirituality, accountability, etc. We now offer one-to-one, small-group 'defuse' reflection groups and retreat days as a part of our portfolio of staff support.

5. Celebrating and championing diversity

We can lament how difficult healthcare has sometimes become because of the multicultural context many of us find ourselves in or we can celebrate diversity. The chaplaincy team firmly believe that when religious care is deemed to be important enough to be an integral part of care then this championing of diversity enhances patient care and wellbeing.

Multifaith not interfaith: not one size fits all

I have found that some folks assume that it is appropriate or helpful to join all the religions together for one provision. My experience as a chaplain is that many families and patients want faith-appropriate care and I believe that out of respect for patients and their needs this is what we should be offering. It is important therefore that staff have training and understand how different faith groups approach end of life and other issues impacted by healthcare. However, you do not need to be of the same faith as the person to offer appropriate religious care. If you are uncomfortable with knowing how to deliver some element of religious care then draw on the specialist resources that are available through chaplaincy or the community. An example of what we do to provide bespoke bereavement services is to offer families both a Christian memorial service and a pastoral/spiritual care walk and picnic at the National Memorial Arboretum, where we have the riverside walk dedicated to our children. Most other faiths do not have a culture of remembering their deceased family members on an arbitrary date.

Individual and personal care: expect a casserole not a roast

Although I am advocating treating individual faiths as separate entities and not assuming a one size fits all, we cannot expect a young person, child or staff member of any one faith to be monochrome, to just be all orthodox, uniformly Christian or Hindu, for example. We have all been influenced by traditions other than our own and by our culture. As with every element of our personality, we all have our own unique way of believing and practising our faith. I use a couple of different images when I talk about this. When approaching a young person or family I tend to expect a casserole, not a roast. What do I mean? A piece of roast meat is an entity in itself, it is the same all the way through – this is sometimes how faith is taught – Christians or Hindus believe this. A casserole, or if you prefer, a fruit smoothie (rather than a fruit bowl) contains lots of different things – it is usually different every time you make it. In reality, families are more like this – they have a faith but the combination of what they believe and how they practise it is uniquely theirs and different from what may be taught on a course or read in a book. Thus each individual or family needs to be seen as a new opportunity to offer spiritual or religious care, and this care should be specific to this particular family or individual to meet their needs, not the last individual or family's needs.

PC: personal care not political correctness

I am not a great fan of political correctness for its own sake. I am in favour of treating people with fairness and justice. Political correctness's motivation could be understood to be exactly that, political not personal. BCH has a Christian chapel, Muslim prayer room and a meditation room for all other faiths and none. This room is intentionally simple and plain so as not to have any images or pictures that could offend or be distracting. It is felt, under equal opportunity policy, that this room should be provided, and rightly so. But what is the reality? Our current Hindu and Sikh chaplains prefer to use the chapel for events. Many of our patients and families will use whatever faith room they want. We will often find prayers from Muslim, Sikh and Hindu children in our prayer book in the chapel. We cannot box people or tell them where and how to worship. Taking some of the objectives of the assessment tools in Chapter 10 will help us to do this, and provide a high-class personal care directed service.

Equal opportunity is not treating everyone the same

It is giving every child and family equal opportunity for care. Why send bereavement anniversary cards to those who believe in reincarnation if they believe this remembering holds their loved one back from their next life? I want each faith service provision to be true to itself and distinctive. Being informed, asking individual families and patients helps us achieve this. We hope the six faith chapters in this book will help to facilitate such care.

The big diversity issues

Health and palliative care are conducive places to engage with some of the big questions and concerns about what it means to work and live in diverse, multifaith and multicultural communities and countries. We have a wonderful opportunity to model all that is good about the potential of multiculturalism:

- communication and language issues, including gestures and touch
- deference
- institutional racism
- colour blindness
- stereotyping
- assumptions
- different understandings of health, illness and death
- we are all from different cultures; even white British people
- we are first and foremost fellow human beings
- understanding demographics is only part of the picture
- we are all essentially ethnocentric.

Underbelly: Understanding and appreciating uniqueness

Unless I really do appreciate and value other faiths and beliefs than my own, I cannot celebrate or champion diversity. This means treating everyone as unique individuals, without assumption or boxing. But it is vital that we continue to promote the importance of such a culture, if we believe 'cultural influences have a significant impact on such health-promoting factors as diet, exercise, and stress-management'.[12]

Learning from other faiths

I observe generosity and graciousness being offered every time I see a man offer a Muslim woman a handshake, and she takes it. My attitude has changed over time about who and what I could learn from whom. I have realized, members from other faiths have inspired me to be a better Christian. One member of staff offered back some of their first salary as a gift to God; the place they chose to do this was on the altar in the chapel, although they were not Christian.

The multifaith religious care team

As the leader of a multifaith team with a religious agenda (as opposed to one within a more normal working environment) we have a unique role within the hospital. There are some elements I have identified, which it is important for those of us responsible for delivering religious and spiritual care to reflect on and consider:

- the necessity of modelling what we teach

- my team members are there because of their faith

- individual members are there to support and facilitate patients and staff's own faith

- with cross-faith referrals there is a need for information for more than just our faith

- we are overt role models – we are representatives of our faith in the hospital in the way that others are not

- the more fundamental a person is in their own faith, the more potential clashes there might be with other staff or practices

- there is an expectation that we may need to set aside some of our personal faith principles for the greater good of the team and the institution.

Part of the feedback we had on the 2014 BBC Two series of our work *Children's Hospital: The Chaplains* was that the public were impressed by how a chaplain of one faith treated, and related to, a child and family of a different faith.

Conclusion

This is an evolving model and I am sharing these values within our hospital and will seek to practise and refine them over time. In seeking to implement effective multifaith care it is crucial to have thought through what your own beliefs and principles are in relation to the issues raised in this chapter.

Notes

1   Spiers, R (2010) 'It's that time of year.' *Wider World Magazine*, December, p.7. Available at https://www.presbyterianireland.org/getmedia/ab4a88d7-41a6-43a2-adf0-3759f28bf69a/its-that-time-of-year.pdf.aspx, accessed 13 January 2015. It is based on Eisely, L. (1969) 'The Star Thrower.' *The Unexpected Universe*. New York: Harcourt, Brace & World.

2   Nash, P., Darby, K. and Nash, S. (2013) 'The spiritual care of sick children: Reflections from a participation project.' *International Journal of Children's Spirituality 18*, 2, 148–161.

3   Darby, K., Nash, P. and Nash, S. (2014) 'Spiritual and religious needs of young people with cancer.' *Cancer Nursing Practice 13*, 2, 32–37.

4   See Paul Nash (2011) *Supporting Dying Children and Their Families*. London: SPCK for further details on the whirlpool of grief.

5   A multidisciplinary team runs the Celebrate Project, which arranges activities for various religious and cultural festivals throughout the year. It is funded by BCH Charities.

6   This has been written up by Paul Nash in Peter Gilbert (ed.) (2013) *Spirituality and End of Life Care*. Hove: Pavilion.

7   Austin, L.J. (2006) 'Spiritual assessment: A chaplain's perspective.' *Explore 2*, 6, 540–542.

8   This is a succinct overview of the choices: www.hss.cmu.edu/philosophy/london/Twins.pdf

9   Sewell, H. (2009) *Working with Ethnicity, Race and Culture in Mental Health*. London: Jessica Kingsley Publishers, p.78.

10   Kub, J.E., Nolan, M.T., Hughes, M.T., Terry, P.T., Sulmasy, D.P., Astrow, A., and Forman, J.H. (2003) 'Religious Importance and Practices of Patients With a Life-Threatening Illness: Implications for Screening Procols.' *Applied Nursing Research 16*, 3, 196–200, p.196.

11   Adair, J. (2002) *Inspiring Leadership*. London: Thorogood, p.57.

12   Andrews, M.M. and Boyle, J.S. (2003) *Transcultural Concepts in Nursing Care*. 4th edn. Philadelphia: Lippincott, Williams and Wilkins, p.345.

2

CARE OF A BUDDHIST CHILD AND FAMILY

Keith Munnings and Madeleine Parkes[1]

Introduction to Buddhism

Buddhism has existed as a spiritual way of life for over 2600 years. Buddhism spread from its origins in India across Asia and today is established in most major continents with an increasing number of followers in Europe, the USA and Australasia. In common with other world religions Buddhism is vast and rich in ideas, so attempts to generalize beliefs and standardize practices can cause problems. However, there are shared common principles that identify an individual as a Buddhist and these can be worked with to support followers and members of different Buddhist communities.

> ### 21ST-CENTURY BUDDHISM
>
> We need to be 21st-century Buddhists. Buddhist practice is to use our intelligence to the maximum to transform our emotions. For this, knowledge is very important. Western scholars often suggest that Buddhism is not so much a religion, but more a science of the mind. (Dalai Lama)[2]

Buddhist denominations may be characterized by the different ways people meditate and how their beliefs affect their daily actions. There are many different types of Buddhism and, where practical and relevant, the differences between them will be accommodated.

Because Buddhism can be seen as a philosophy on life, which evolved over time within different cultures, there are very few rules and doctrines around family life and roles that are purely faith driven.

Therefore many Buddhists adopt secular or cultural views concerning the roles and expectations of women and men, the responsibilities of children and care of the family. For this reason the information provided below on culture, religion and spirituality should be taken as a starting point, from where you can be made aware of some of the differences you may encounter. However, the golden rule always applies, no matter how much factual knowledge you have read – *ask, don't assume, what the individual wishes at the time to be paramount.*

Beliefs and rituals

Buddhists take refuge in the 'Three Jewels'. In the same way as precious gems may be treasured, taking refuge is paying the deepest respect to the Buddha, *dharma* (*dhamma*) and *sangha*, and primarily relying upon these jewels during life. Buddha refers to the founder of Buddhism (mind). *Dharma* refers to Buddha's teachings and the practice of them (voice). *Sangha* is the Buddhist community (body), which practises *dharma* and helps others to do the same. Buddhists may also have a spiritual guide who they consider to be the main representative of the Three Jewels for them and upon whom they rely for spiritual and religious guidance.

The 'Four Noble Truths' can help us to understand all the teachings of the Buddha. The human being who became 'the Buddha' by attaining full enlightenment experienced these truths – of suffering, its cause, its cessation and the paths leading to its cessation – and shared these truths with others.

Buddhists believe that the body and mind are two separate continuums and that the mind lives in the body temporarily before it permanently leaves the body at the time of death to go to future lives. Buddhists understand that their mind or consciousness will follow different paths in accordance with the type of action they create and what seeds, virtuous or otherwise, ripen at the time of death. *Karma* is a Sanskrit word meaning 'action' and gives the Buddhist the opportunity to accept and understand how difficulties and suffering are the effect and result of previous actions and intentions, generated both in this life and in previous lives. In order to become liberated from this suffering, Buddhists work to purify negative imprints on their mental continuum, reduce and eradicate negative states of mind, and increase and familiarize themselves with pure and positive states of mind. They do this for the benefit of everyone, not just for themselves, and believe this is the way to true happiness.

Meditation is part of a Buddhist way of life. It helps increase faith in Buddha, helps the *sangha* (community) to practise *dharma* and helps to deepen understanding of Buddha's teachings. Buddhist practice aims at purifying any negativity from the mind and increasing good fortune and benefit for the self and others. Buddhists believe that by relying upon Buddha with strong faith, practising *dharma* sincerely, and relying on their *sangha* friends and spiritual guides, they can attain liberation from '*samsara*' (the cycle of uncontrolled rebirth). As long as their mind remains uncontrolled, they experience without choice, life after life, the cycle and sufferings of *samsara*.

Denominations

Theravada Buddhism is often called 'southern Buddhism' because it is mostly followed in Sri Lanka, Myanmar (Burma), Thailand, Laos and Cambodia. In Pali, Theravada means 'the Way of the Elders'.

Mahayana Buddhism is found mainly in north Asia and the Far East. They share basic teachings but are very distinct from each other. Mahayana includes schools of Zen (Vietnamese, Japanese Soto, Japanese Rinse and Korean), Chan, Pureland and a group of Japanese Lotus *Sutra* schools.

Vajrayana Buddhism is mainly Tibetan and includes Kagyu, Gelug, Nyingma and Sakya lineages. Kadampa Buddhists do not mix religious practices with any political, cultural or national concerns in order to practise Buddha's teachings clearly.

Cultural influences are large in Buddhism. For example, Chinese Buddhists have different funeral rites to others, sometimes lasting up to 49 days. A Thai Buddhist family may pour water on the deceased's head as an act of purity. In Tibet it is believed that the deceased person doesn't know they are dead for four days and yet the monk's chants can still reach them.

Historical events and holy books

Born Prince Siddhartha Guatama, Lord Buddha's early life was one of luxury. He was protected from and had never experienced any grief, sorrow or misery. On a number of different days, while visiting a park, he saw an old man, a sick man, a corpse and a monk, none of whom he had ever seen before. He realized for himself that he, as well as all beings, would in time be subject to birth, ageing, sickness and death – only the monk appeared to him to be calm and at peace. He realized the impermanence of everything and with that motivation he decided to forsake this opulent worldly life and search for the truth.

The term 'Buddha' means 'awakened one', one who has completely abandoned all delusions and their imprints, and refers to someone who has awoken from the sleep of ignorance and understands the way things truly exist. The founder of Buddhism, Buddha Shakyamuni, is usually the person people refer to as 'the Buddha'. The Buddha demonstrated the ultimate goal of supreme inner peace, full enlightenment, at Bodh Gaya in India in 589 BCE (before the common era).

Buddha was asked to teach *dharma* and gave 84,000 teachings in three main phases. Buddhism developed throughout many countries in the world and the teachings were made suitable for people of that time and that place, which is why the traditions are so rich in diversity. Development continues today with different traditions welcoming people to listen to *dharma*. Buddhism has many holy books and texts, including Buddha's *sutra* and *tantra* and teachings. The texts that a person would rely upon would be those written in a way that is familiar with their tradition/denomination.

Names and greetings

When naming a baby, Buddhist parents may choose a name that is tied to the day, month or season that the child is born, in line with the traditional practice of consulting astrological charts to influence the name choice. Historically, baby-naming ceremonies were considered secular affairs by most Buddhist traditions and therefore may not be widely practised today. Babies can be named after teachers or persons from within a tradition or to reflect a link to a specific Buddhist practice or *bodhisattva* role model.

Family life

In the past, monastic Buddhism appealed to single adults who were interested in pursuing enlightenment, which required great levels of solitude and discipline. Early Buddhism emphasized celibacy and separateness, as having relationships and fulfilling family responsibilities creates earthly attachments, which some Buddhists would see as a hindrance to detaching from material life in order to focus on the spiritual. Because of these early foundations, many Buddhists may adopt secular or cultural views of the roles of women, the responsibilities of children and the role of family. In some traditions young boys could enter a monastery as a novice monk from as young as four years old, when they were deemed old enough to be educated and not dependent upon their mother for their daily needs. Cultural influences of gender and family roles will have an impact. For example, within many Asian Buddhist cultures this typically translates into a traditional, patriarchal family structure with clearly defined familial roles.

Buddhism does not restrict either the educational opportunities of women or their religious freedom. The Buddha unhesitatingly accepted that women are capable of realizing the Truth, just as men are. Emanations of Buddha in female aspect are not considered inferior to male, and there are examples in scripture of Buddha's choosing the female form as a positive choice. Buddhist ethics emphasize that the role of husbands and wives are to cultivate respect and faithfulness to one another and to build a mutually supported, peaceful environment within the home.

WOMEN IN FAMILY LIFE

Buddhism does not consider women as being inferior to men. Buddhism, while accepting the biological and physical differences between the two sexes, considers men and women to be equally useful to society.

Parents can share Buddhist teachings and practice with their children, and often lead by example by practising Buddhism and living out Buddhist values as a way of teaching their children. Parents may involve their children in the *sangha*, or religious community, and often classes are offered for children at many Buddhist centres and during festivals.

In many Buddhist homes there will be a small shrine with a statue of the Buddha on display. The statue could be one of many forms of the Buddha depending on the tradition or school of Buddhism that is followed. The shrine is a focal point of the religious practice of the family and these shrines will have incense, candles and flowers decorating them. Individuals may then undertake personal prayers or devotions, which can include parents praying with their younger children. Some children may attend Buddhist schools and could be involved in faith practices with their teachers and school friends.

Languages

Buddhism is a worldwide religion and adherents will speak a wide variety of languages. The Buddha gave no preference for any particular language.

Stories and attitudes to children

History tells us the story of Guatama Buddha leaving his wife and son in order to seek a path to awakening. Traditionally there has been an emphasis on celibacy and separateness in many but not all Buddhist traditions. As Buddhism has become established across the world, Buddhist positions on children and childhood have emerged.

Images of 'mother' and examples of unconditional enduring love for her child are used to illustrate the Buddha's love for all beings in traditional Buddhist literature. Similarly, in Mahayana Buddhism, meditating on the role of the mother and the love she generates for her child is used to support the tradition of the *bodhisattva* (someone who has developed great compassion and who wishes to become liberated in order to save others from suffering).

BUDDHISM AND CHILDREN

Buddhism, by and large, has little to say about children directly. Likewise child directed rituals are few: there are no birth-purification rites or infant baptisms, nor are there rites on circumcision or even clear rulings on childrearing...nonetheless we can find a range of fascinating child-related issues in the vast corpus of Buddhist writing and practice.[3]

Children are respected very much, just as any person would be. Depending on their tradition, they may have various meditations, practices and studies in which they engage. For many Buddhist families, children are likely to be taught Buddhist beliefs naturally through their parents' example. The child would be allowed to choose their own faith, if they wish to follow one; it would not be forced upon them.

Across different Buddhist traditions, bodhisattvas are those who have followed the path of Buddhism to the point of enlightenment but then elected to stay on earth to help the suffering of others. Bodhisattvas such as Guanyin (Taiwanese Buddhism) and Dizang (Chinese Buddhism) are said to grant fertility to men and women. In Japanese Buddhism, Jizo, another *bodhisattva*, is considered the special guardian of deceased children as well as protecting those who are alive.

Children and adults are viewed as equal on the premise that childhood is a stage, a part of developing in this lifetime, but the person's true experience is unknown to us and all genders are equal according to the teachings of the Buddha.

Care of Buddhist patients and their families in hospital

Buddhists will be different in their beliefs and practices depending upon their tradition and circumstances, so the information given here should be seen as a guide from which to ask further questions. Not every Buddhist is in a Buddhist family. Some Buddhist families have other faiths within them and not every member of the same family will follow the same rules and ideas, so the golden rule of *ask, don't assume* is paramount. Key learning points include:

- There are many traditions within all world faiths and Buddhism is no different. Although all follow the same core tenets and beliefs, practices will vary.

- A peaceful environment to allow meditation would be important to a Buddhist patient and family.

- Having images of Buddha, small statutes or ritual objects can bring support and comfort.

- Mantras, prayers, music and chants all form part of Buddhist practice, and the child/family may appreciate time and space to perform these.

- Follow personal family wishes at all times, but remember these may be conflicting.

- Children should be respected and conversed with in a non-patronizing way.

A CHAPLAIN'S VIEW

We were caring for the parents of a baby who had been born with a digestive tract problem and was not likely to survive for more than ten days. The parents, who were Sri Lankan, had been living in Britain for two years and had very little support from family and friends, who were all still in Sri Lanka. Even the Sri Lankan Buddhist Temple was over half an hour away.

The parents chose to spend a few hours away from the hospital visiting the temple, offering prayers and speaking to the monk. Ward staff were surprised that they would leave their baby son at such a critical time, but as Buddhist chaplains we were able to explain this and the importance of faith for the family, even if our own understanding was more of the head than the heart.

We offered our presence to the couple, as fellow Buddhists, which was welcomed. We also chanted in Pali around the cot of this little boy. It meant a lot to the parents, and later that day the Sri Lankan monk came to offer his support too. We were able to offer ourselves as a resource; even though our backgrounds were different, the resources we used (chants) were part of the same faith.

Food and prohibited products

Some Buddhists are vegetarians, based on the principle of the first precept, a teaching about being responsible for not killing other beings. However, Buddha himself was not a vegetarian and he did not teach vegetarianism. Vegetarian practices differ widely across different Buddhist schools and cultures. For example, Mahayana Buddhism in China emphasizes being vegetarian but both the monks and laymen/laywomen of the Mahayana tradition in Japan and Tibet usually eat meat. For some, eating can be a primary spiritual practice but the rituals may be subtle and not easily observed. The family may bring food from home for the child in hospital. A child may not be eating hospital food for reasons other than illness, such as not liking the taste of hospital food or not being used to the flavours. Buddhist patients and families may observe festivals throughout the year and certain fasts (sometimes not eating after midday), which will affect dietary needs.

Modesty and hygiene

Care provided by staff of the same gender is preferable for teenagers and young adults, in order to preserve modesty. This isn't required for children who have not reached puberty, although ideas about modesty may be strong, and even young children may not want to change in front of others. Buddhist children may prefer to shower under running water, which is preferred over a bath in some cultures. Families and children from a range of cultural backgrounds may eat with their hands, often the right hand. There is a high regard for purity, both physical and spiritual, so washing may occur very frequently, especially before consuming food.

Children and teenagers from immigrant families may have a mixed identity around dress and language. Traditional dress may be worn, as well as Western clothes. Religious symbols worn on the body as jewellery, such as *vajras* or images of Buddha, should be left in place wherever possible. Any threads or beads around a child's wrist, chest or neck should be respected as a religious symbol and should not be removed without consultation. Information should be provided to staff in other treatment areas, especially theatres, so they can make any reasonable adjustments.

Taboos

Displaying the sole of the foot is taboo in some countries that have high Buddhist populations. Pointing the feet towards a statue of the Buddha can be seen as disrespectful, as the feet are considered the lowest and most impure part of the body. Placing *dharma* objects, books and texts on the floor or stepping over them is disrespectful and should be avoided. In some traditions, placing *dharma* objects below the waist is considered incorrect. Some Buddhists are uncomfortable with the recent trade in objects for the home representing parts of the Buddha's body (e.g. Buddha hand candle holders). It is always best to ask and get clarification; what matters to some is less important to others.

More generally, the whole area of taboos and what may or may not be spoken about by a Buddhist family reaffirms the need for sensitivity towards the diversity of cultural differences found across Buddhism.

By the bedside

Items that a child in hospital may have by their bed include whatever the individual and the family would find most beneficial in helping to create a positive and peaceful environment. In some cases, images of Buddhas would be present. Viewing or visualizing an image of Buddha and recognizing his extraordinary good qualities enables Buddhists to receive blessings, which transform the mind from a weak state into a positive state and from a disturbed state into a peaceful state. A sick child may wish to practise their faith in hospital. They may try to focus on loving others and other practices to help make their experience meaningful. This would depend upon their capacity and there would certainly not be any expectation that they should practise in any particular way. For younger children, brightly coloured picture books telling the story of Buddha or showing images of Buddha are available and can help calm the mind and move attention to a more positive object, but these should be offered only after consultation with the family.

The popular Tibetan chant *Om mani padme hum* may bring a sense of peace as it brings to mind the embodiment of compassion. A useful text, accessible to Buddhists of all traditions, is the *Dhammapada* – there are many versions available. It comprises a number of verses that can be reflected upon one at a time and provide good 'food for thought'.

Specific religious and cultural needs

- A translator may be needed as Buddhist families may speak Cantonese, Mandarin, Japanese, Thai, Burmese, Sri Lankan and many other languages.

- Every effort should be made to use a professional translator, not a family member of the patient. Where practical, a chaplain may be able to offer translation skills depending on organizational policy.

- If using a family member to translate, be very mindful that they are hearing the news you are telling them for the first time and may not fully understand what is being said. If they do understand, they may not be able to find the most accurate words to translate the information – this is particularly true for unfamiliar medical terminology or concepts – and they should be invited to clarify their understanding with you.

- A spiritual friend, Buddhist teacher, monk or nun from their Buddhist tradition could be invited to support the child and their family and friends. This may need to be suggested to the family, who may not know this is an option for them.

Age-specific considerations

Babies

In some traditional cultures, monks are invited after birth to bless the baby and chant. Within one month of birth the baby may be brought to the *vihara*, or temple, and presented near a Buddha statue. Arising in the 1970s, there is now a tradition in some Japanese and Taiwanese Buddhist cultures to offer rituals for foetuses. A Buddhist chaplain working with stillbirth and aborted foetuses may offer blessings and rituals around this. There are no religious considerations about breast-feeding although there may be cultural ones, depending on the cultural background of the family.

Infants

When weaning infants on to solid food, consider if they should be fed vegetarian food and with what restrictions, according to family wishes. Nutritional guidelines and policies should be considered and discussed, especially if the child is unwell. Be aware of any white or red threads tied around the infant's wrist, neck or chest, and do not remove them without permission. It is important to view these threads as expressions of love and concern for the child's wellbeing; they are not just decorations.

Children and teenagers

Parents are encouraged to teach their children to be compassionate and responsible, although in many traditions there is no formal requirement to raise children with strict Buddhist teachings. Often teachings are fully integrated into family life and behavioural expectations, so the child/young person may not view themselves or their parents as particularly religious, but they may become distressed if something they instinctively accept and believe in is challenged or overlooked. There are no specific religious requirements for children; however, there will be familial, and possibly tradition- and faith-community-based and cultural expectations on older children and teenagers.

Working with the family

This can be a very rewarding experience for all involved. It is useful to have some basic understanding of family dynamics as they apply to diverse family units before starting to consider what is specifically faith- and belief-based.

Conducive environment

This would preferably be a quiet space, possibly suitable for meditation and reflection. However, it is unlikely that lack of such facilities would cause offence. Rather, the desirability of quiet may help prepare for a peaceful death. Allowing some degree of privacy is usually appreciated and can help reduce stress.

Views of suffering

Buddhists do not believe that suffering is imposed on them from outside, nor do they believe that they will be judged for their actions. They believe that their own actions determine their future experiences in both this and future lives – cause and effect, the Law of *Karma*. It is therefore their personal responsibility, with Buddha's blessings and the support of the *sangha*, to apply *dharma* wisdom to their minds so that throughout this life, at the time of death and in future lives, they will create happiness and freedom for themselves and others.

Some people misunderstand the teachings on *karma*, thinking that these teachings suggest that a person's suffering is their fault. This is not the case. A person creates the causes (*karma*) for suffering because they are suffering from negative states of mind. Therefore, it is acting under negative states of mind that is the cause and never the fault of the person themselves. The true nature of every living being is kindness and purity, and we only engage in harmful actions because we are like a sick person who is confused and is not seeing things clearly. It is never appropriate to blame a person for creating the causes of suffering because nobody would intentionally create the causes of suffering which are described as desire-based – for example, wanting things to be different from what they are. Buddha's teachings are clear that seeing fault in others is not beneficial; seeing our own shortcomings and making changes to our own mind are. By removing this confusion from our minds and by learning to see things clearly, as they really are, we can free ourselves from our negative states of mind, and our true nature, our Buddha nature, will gradually become manifest.

Learning to accept that death is an entirely natural and inevitable part of life is core to Buddhist beliefs. There is unlikely to be a tendency to try to hide what is happening amongst the wider community and indeed practitioners would be encouraged to make prayers for the dying person. You may hear terms used such as 'my death time' or 'our child's death time'. Do not confuse this acceptance of death as a natural part of the wheel of life, as meaning Buddhists do not love their families or experience loss and bereavement; it may just be expressed in a way you are unfamiliar with. Some Buddhists will find the loss of a child a major test of their personal faith.

Attitudes to medical care

Buddhists generally have a positive attitude to medical care. Buddhists would appreciate direct and honest communication from the medical staff, in line with their core belief in 'right speech'. Buddhist ethics around medical decisions are still developing and therefore the family may wish to seek religious advice or support when medical decisions need to be made.

Understanding illness and disease

Buddha taught in the Four Noble Truths that while we are confused about the true nature of things, we experience what is known as 'samsara' and our lives are pervaded by suffering. All living beings in samsara, without exception, have to experience the sufferings of birth, sickness, ageing and death, having to part with what they like, having to encounter what they do not like and failing to satisfy their desires. It is because we have the good fortune to have a precious human body that we also have the potential to experience the sufferings of the human body. Particular sufferings are caused by previous actions, or *karma*, which we engaged in because of our confused minds, such as anger, jealousy and other negative minds. *Karma* is universal and is a mystical concept – it is not simple to understand and apply to suffering. The general concept is that at every moment in life we have the opportunity to be present and act responsibly, which impacts our future both in this life and the next.

The concept of *karma* does not mean that disease is a person's fault. Quite the opposite. The real object of blame is our negative states of mind, such as anger, which impel us to create the causes for suffering. There is a view in some Buddhist traditions that a child has not developed enough to work with *dharma*, or Buddhist teaching, and this can have an impact on views about how much *karma* is responsible for the current illness.

A Buddhist practitioner would apply effort to view suffering as an opportunity, but this may be very difficult for a younger child, experiencing pain for example. Experiencing suffering may teach a Buddhist to develop the wish to reduce and eventually abandon the causes of suffering. This can be done by overcoming negative states of mind by going for refuge to Buddha, *dharma* (the practice of Buddha's teachings) and *sangha* (community, or spiritual friends). Specific methods of meditation and mindfulness, or focusing on *dharma* objects could help a child or young person to focus away from their suffering towards a more peaceful and rested state, and families may want the opportunity to help them to do this rather than reliance on more accepted medical practices.

OFFERING EXPLANATIONS – A CHAPLAIN'S VIEW

When asked to offer an explanation for why a child may suffer and die, I wouldn't want to offer one specific view. This is not because there isn't a Buddhist understanding of suffering and death, but because it is more important to be offering compassion and wisdom than theoretical explanations. These can come later but pastoral care based on kindness and compassion, a key part of Buddhist belief and practice, is what will be remembered and be most helpful.

Understanding mental illness

From a Buddhist perspective, mental illness is caused by negative states of mind, otherwise known as delusions. All living beings suffer from delusions such as ignorance, selfishness, craving, anger, jealousy, but for some individuals these tendencies are stronger than they are for others. Delusions cause us all to act in unpredictable and often irrational ways. Mental ill health is within this same continuum but rather more severe in its presentation. What states of mind we experience depend upon the mental habits we have brought with us from previous lives and what causes these to arise for us in this life. For as long as living beings suffer from negative states of mind, suffering is inevitable. Therefore, it is never appropriate to blame any person for their suffering.

A CHAPLAIN'S VIEW

It is clear that the teachings and practices found in Buddhism have much to contribute to mental health. There is such a wealth and richness of teaching on the cultivation of a wholesome mind and mental states.

My personal experience of working with patients has been one of being cautious and wary – I do not want to be acting in any way that contradicts or interferes with a patient's existing programme of treatment, whether this be about their prescribed medication or any other therapeutic approach mental health services are providing.

As a Buddhist chaplain, through mindfulness practices and by deep listening to the patient expressing their needs, I may help explore and find a 'middle way' through the 'roller-coaster' of emotion arising from their struggles and successes.

Pain management

Buddhist practice encourages 'staying with' pain and suffering; the act of resisting pain can often make it worse. Mindful acceptance of pain can actually diminish pain, and might even get rid of it completely. Mindfulness meditation enables the raw sensations of pain to be explored until you begin to accept them. Some Buddhists might call out to the Buddha, similar to practitioners of other religious faiths who call out to God. Some take refuge in the Buddha during times of pain and difficulty, others will respectfully prostrate, putting their hands together at their heart. This is not to diminish the experience of pain but rather to bring to mind a spiritual understanding of reality that may shift the perspective of the current moment to a more spacious place. Most Buddhists would not request the Buddha to intervene, rather they would draw strength from Buddha, *dharma* or *sangha* reminding them of a spiritual understanding of pain and suffering during this time.

Being present, sitting with pain without trying to fix it or change it, can be an important practice for many Buddhists as it helps face the realities of human nature and understand them better. While being present and mindful of pain and suffering, emotions such as anger, blame and disbelief may arise. Working with pain through love and compassion helps to provide relief from anxiety and better focus the mind. In Buddhism these processes always start with kindness towards oneself and lead on to a greater empathy for others.

Mindfulness practices for children have been developed and some schools are embracing mindfulness as a valuable addition to the daily life of young people. The family may already practise some form of meditation in daily life. Supportive prayers and focusing on specific Buddha images can help younger children to manage their pain, as can chanting mantras or visits from ordained *sangha*. The issue of analgesia will need to be explored with the child and the family, some parents would find the administration of strong analgesia to their child challenging and may not wish to give consent. Working with the family is of paramount importance in such situations.

Traditional healing and medicine

There will be significant cultural influences on the views of traditional healing and medicine. Across many cultures there are many systems of traditional medicine that involve the use of herbs and plants, changes in diet and the prescription of yoga, meditation or spiritual treatments.

There is also the influence of Tibetan traditional healing systems (which includes psychiatry), which has superficial similarities to Indian *Ayurveda* medicine. It is practised alongside Buddhism but has its own philosophies and ideas.[4]

Understanding death

Buddhists believe that death is inescapable and the timing is uncertain. As Buddhists recognize that life is impermanent, always changing and things never stay the same for long, death is an accepted part of life. However, most traditions accept that this human life is precious as it allows us to study and experience *dharma*. So, as much as possible is done to extend the length of life and avoid untimely death. Many Buddhists believe that the body and mind are separate, and it is understood that the mind, or consciousness, moves on to a different life at death but the form of body is left behind. Uncontrolled death is part of the endless rebirth cycle known as *samsara*, or more colloquially, reincarnation.

Because of an emphasis on reality and its acceptance, Buddhist families may have talked to their children about death extensively in order to remove any taboo or fears about it. Children are often very aware of death, particularly if they have been in hospital and made friends with other children on the ward who have died. They may have many questions and worries. Buddhists may openly discuss their beliefs about death in an age-appropriate way with their children. Death will be part of the Buddhist family understanding even if it is not often formally discussed.

> **DEATH AS UNIVERSAL**
>
> From a famous tale:
>
> Kisa Gotami, having lost her child, becomes inconsolable and carries the dead child around until the Buddha promises to revive the child if Kisa Gotami will collect mustard seeds from every family that hasn't had a death in the family. In the course of trying to find these mustard seeds, she comes to realise how universal death is and joins the Buddhist order.[5]

Despite this, there is an understanding that untimely and premature deaths are still difficult to acknowledge and cope with. Buddhists may try to focus on the positive 'ripples' that can arise from a tragic death – valuing the preciousness of all human birth, however short the actual life. Some parents have founded a charitable fund in memory of their lost child – and thereby unfortunate circumstances ultimately can do good for humanity. This does not negate the strength of emotion and loss for the family and community.

Preparing for death

In Buddhism a 'good' death is one that has been prepared for as part of life's journey. The state of the mind immediately before death is believed to have a significant effect on the nature of the person's reincarnation, so for Buddhists a peaceful mind, removed of fear and desire, is important at the time of death. This may be dependent on the personality of the person dying, which is why Buddhists may wish to cultivate an accepting attitude to death throughout life in order to prepare for their final moments.

Hospital staff and volunteers can contribute to this 'good death' by providing a peaceful and calm environment, by offering emotional support to the patient and family/ friends in order to alleviate worry and fear. Buddhists would reject criteria for death that are based solely on loss of consciousness or higher brain functioning. For example, a child in a permanent vegetative state would still require constant care from a Buddhist perspective, otherwise this would be considered killing. Some Buddhist traditions (that have established medicine systems within them) have methods for recognizing signs that death is approaching. Families may already be looking for evidence of these signs or could be informed of these by members of their *sangha*. These signs are viewed as positive because they give people time to prepare. Chaplains are well placed to explain the significance of these signs to hospital staff who may not understand or accept the concept or the effect on the child or family.

> **A CHAPLAIN'S VIEW**
>
> Death is not a taboo for practising Buddhists, who may have meditated and thought about suffering, illness and death as part of their engagement with Buddhist philosophy. Preparing for death can be done 'well' by Buddhist families and chaplains. There is a well-known analogy about preparation for death based around the way a wave comes to the shore: once it has begun to build it has its own momentum and you can try to resist or work with it.

Meditation practices, including simple ones that focus on in-and-out breathing or reciting 'let go' can be used to focus the mind, relax the body and calm the emotions. Children respond well to some meditation practices and may already be familiar with them if the family has taught them. Use of guided visualizations can help children to develop a happy mind, by focusing on Buddha or peaceful places.

Variations in preparing for death

Culture and ethnicity are influential factors in the practice of Buddhism. Typically, Western Buddhists will blend their medical and scientific explanations of illness and death, and may have more flexibility with death customs and rituals that are not necessarily Buddhist. Chinese Buddhists often revert to very traditional and specific Buddhist practices and rituals, even if they are not actively practising Buddhists.

Buddhists who have moved from overseas to live in the UK often have very specific religious customs that are used at the time of death and beyond. Traditionally, these involved Buddhist monks visiting regularly and performing most of the rites and rituals, which is unlikely to happen with such frequency in the West.

When a child is approaching death:

- A quiet and peaceful environment should be created (as far as this is possible).

- The family should be kept closely informed as religious practices may need to be completed.

- The family may wish to chant and/or say prayers as this is believed to relieve pain; space and time should be given for this.

- If the child is conscious, they may wish to recite some mantras or chants if they are familiar with them. If the child is unconscious, this responsibility rests with the family.

- The child may or may not be familiar with Buddhist practices, depending on the family's own practices and beliefs about raising children in a religion. If the child does not have a strong Buddhist faith, it may be helpful to remind them of positive things they have done in their life, or of positive qualities such as love and compassion and kindness, instead of formal religious rituals. A chaplain can help to navigate the family's and patient's wishes.

- 'The basic aim is to avoid any objects or people that generate strong attachment or anger in the mind of the dying person.'[6]

- In some traditions, during the last hours/moments, the child's body should not be touched other than at the crown of the head. Medical monitoring procedures should be limited.

Immediately after death:

- Sutras or longer texts/chants and practices for those who have recently died may be recited at the time leading up to and immediately after death.

- In many Buddhist traditions, the body should not be touched for as long as possible. Traditionally, this was several days although realistically in hospital a few hours may suffice.

- The eyes are closed and last offices can be performed.

Organ donation and post-mortem

Organ and tissue donation would be a personal choice and should not be assumed. Buddhists believe that the consciousness can take time to leave the body and that interference with the body could disturb the consciousness and direct it towards future lives of suffering rather than peace and happiness. This is of significant importance and must be considered by transplant coordinators in their conversations with families and individuals. Prayers in accordance with the deceased's Buddhist tradition as soon as possible after death will help to reassure loved ones that the individual's consciousness will be protected as they move on to their future lives. Donation involving older children and young adults could involve conversations with *sangha* and family around gifting organs and tissue for the benefit of others, but such issues should not be pushed or assumed by staff.

Hospice care

Buddhist families would not have any reservations about hospice care, and there are some Buddhist organizations that work with hospices to provide spiritual support for the dying and the bereaved (for example the Buddhist Hospice Trust). However, some families may not have a good understanding of hospice care because of their culture or background, and the nature of hospice care should be explained.

Caring for the family after the death of their child

After death the family may be visited regularly by Buddhist monks or nuns or lamas, who will offer blessings for the deceased child that are believed to reach them wherever they are now. Support from the wider family and the Buddhist community is traditionally very large and ongoing.

From a Buddhist perspective, it is important to allow feelings from losing a child to surface, such as grief, pain and absence. There is an understanding that the more we can open our hearts to the pain, the quicker the mind can heal and regain its balance. The death of a loved one can also be seen as a transformative period for those left behind, who must learn to live with the loss from a spiritual perspective.

The funeral

Prayers, mantras, recitation of the scriptures and rituals will be conducted by the faith leader or chaplain at a funeral service. Often, presents are offered at a funeral, such as flowers, incense and chanting. The funeral will be a celebration of the life of the recently dead individual. Readings may be offered by family and friends.

Funeral rituals also involve reciting sacred texts. They include other religious practices as well, especially merit transfer ceremonies and may be seen to be designed to bestow additional *karma* upon the dead. There may be times when protective rites exorcise evil influences. In some traditions Buddhist monks may come with the family to the funeral. The family and all their friends offer food and candles to

COMMUNITY RESPONSE TO DEATH – A CHAPLAIN'S EXPERIENCE

When a child died recently within the Kadampa Buddhist community, prayers were made at Buddhist centres and temples across the world. After death, *powa* or 'transference of consciousness' prayers are made and this can offer great comfort to the families and friends of the deceased. It enables the family to believe that the deceased person is no longer suffering but is free from *samsara* and will experience permanent inner peace.

the monks. Goodwill is created by these gifts and it is believed that the goodwill helps the lingering spirit of the dead person.

Cremation is preferred over burial by many Buddhists, and Buddha himself was cremated. However, there is no religious preference and it would be up to the family to decide. Cultural influences would also be present in the decision-making process.

Continuing bonds

Bonds with the child will stay with the family and friends through memories and remembrance. A ritual called *punya tithi* is done every year in some Buddhist traditions on the anniversary of the death, where family and friends come together to remember and offer respects to the deceased.

Key festivals

A widely celebrated festival is that of Vesak (or Wesak or 'Buddha day'), usually on the full moon in May. Buddhists celebrate the birth, enlightenment and final death of the Buddha. Different traditions will celebrate different festivals. For some, 'festival' can mean a Buddhist gathering, shared prayers or empowerment ceremonies. Buddhists have less commonly celebrated festivals than other faiths but *Dharma* day is perhaps the most significant.

Celebrating Dharma *Day*

Dharma Day celebrated the beginning of the Buddha's teaching. In the early years of Buddhism it marked the beginning of the monsoon season which lasted for three months, and during this time Buddha and his followers spent time in meditation and reflection before resuming their travelling, passing on Buddha's teachings. Today it is seen as an opportunity to give thanks to Buddha and other enlightened teachers. Ways of celebrating *Dharma* Day include making bead bracelets which can be used as a tool for reflection; creating a banner to say thank you to those who teach us; and playing musical statues as a way of showing how for Buddhists staying still and reflecting on what they have learnt is very important.

Further reading

Nagaraja, D. (2008) *Buddha at Bedtime: Tales of Love and Wisdom for you to Read with your Child to Enchant, Enlighten and Inspire.* London: Duncan Baird Publishers.

Snel, E. (2013) *Sitting Still like a Frog: Mindfulness Exercises for Kids (and their Parents).* Boston, MA: Shambhala Press.

Notes

1   With particular thanks to Kelsang Leksang and Yve White-Smith for their contributions to this chapter.

2   Gobal Puri, S (2012) 'We need to be 21st century Buddists: Dalai Lama.' *The Times of India,* 28 September. Available at http://articles.timesofindia.indiatimes.com/2012-09-28/india/34146986_1_dalai-lama-buddhism-monasteries, accessed 13 January 2015.

3   Cole, A. (2011) 'Buddhism.' In D.S. Browning and M.J. Bunge (eds) *Children and Childhood in World Religions: Primary Sources and Texts.* New Brunswick, NJ: Rutgers University Press, p.227.

4   International Academy for Traditional Tibetan Medicine. Available at www.iattm.net, accessed on 9 December 2013.

5   Cole, A. (2011) 'Buddhism.' In D.S. Browning and M.J. Bunge (eds) *Children and Childhood in World Religions: Primary Sources and Texts.* New Brunswick: Rutgers University Press, p.283.

6   *The Spiritual Needs of the Dying: A Buddhist Perspective.* Compiled by Ven. Pende Hawter. Available at www.buddhanet.net/spirit_d.htm, accessed on 18 November 2013.

3

CARE OF A CHRISTIAN CHILD AND FAMILY

Paul Nash and Madeleine Parkes[1]

Introduction to Christianity

Christians follow the teachings of Jesus of Nazareth, who lived 2000 years ago. Christianity is one of the three Abrahamic faiths (along with Judaism and Islam) which trace their history to the prophet Abraham, as described in the Hebrew Scriptures (the Christian Old Testament). There are 2 billion Christians worldwide. For many parts of the Western world, Christianity has been influential in shaping culture and spirituality for many hundreds of years, so there will be people who are 'culturally Christian' and understand some of Christianity's teachings and practices without actively being part of a Christian community or church.

> **21ST-CENTURY CHRISTIANITY**
>
> Christianity in the 21st century is a global religion with nearly a third of the world's population as adherents, half of these being Roman Catholics. The influence of Christianity has been seen as declining in the West with regular debates about the impact of secularism. There is also a growing concern about the persecution of Christians in different parts of the world. While the three main traditions of Christianity are Roman Catholic, Protestant and Orthodox there are around 41,000 different denominations across the world.

Beliefs and rituals

Christians believe in one God, a God of supreme love. Jesus Christ is the Son of God, and the promised saviour of humankind. Christians believe that God sent his Son Jesus to earth to save humanity from the consequences of its sins and that eternal life in heaven is available to those who have faith, seek and choose to follow Jesus. Some Christians refer to this as 'the Good News' or 'the gospel'. Jesus' teachings can be summarized briefly as the love of God and love of one's neighbour.

One of the most important concepts in Christianity is that of Jesus giving his life on the Cross (the Crucifixion) and rising from the dead on the third day (the Resurrection). The Christian holy book is the Bible, and consists of the Old and New Testaments. Christian holy days such as Easter and Christmas are important milestones in the Western secular calendar as well as the Christian calendar. Christians also believe in the Holy Spirit, who is the active presence of God on earth. Belief in the devil or a force of evil that works against God (but is never more powerful than God) is part of Christian belief and teaching for some. Additionally, the Holy Spirit is considered the third part of the Godhead or Trinity (the three important figures in Christianity, with God the Father and Jesus the Son making up the other two).

Many Christians will believe in the importance of Holy Communion, which is a church service including the consumption of bread and wine as a symbolic remembrance of Jesus, as commanded in the Bible. Sometimes wine will be substituted with non-alcoholic alternatives such as grape juice. Baptism is an initiation ritual, which in some traditions happens to babies and parents make promises to bring up the child in the Christian faith, or it may not occur until someone makes a personal decision to better follow the teachings of Jesus. Emergency baptisms when a child's life is at risk are a regular feature of chaplaincy, although any baptized person can baptize another if it is an emergency.

Concept of worship in Christianity

Prayer is the means by which Christians communicate with their God. The New Testament records that Jesus taught his disciples how to pray and that he encouraged them to address God as *Father* or *Lord*. Christians believe that they continue this tradition and the Lord's Prayer is often recited. Other personal prayers, including for oneself and others as well as world events, are common. Whilst prayer is often directed to God as Father, Jesus or the Holy Spirit, some traditions encourage prayer to God through intermediaries such as saints and martyrs. A crucifix (image of Christ on the Cross) or a plain cross is seen as a helpful reminder that Christ died, offered himself up, simply out of love for each and every one of us. Candles may be lit as a reminder that Christ is the 'Light of the world'. Hymns and songs are also important parts of Christian worship.

Denominations

Christianity has divided into many denominations over the centuries. Each denomination has its own beliefs and practices, but they are usually considered part of Christianity because they agree on such fundamentals as the Bible, the person of Jesus and the relationship between Jesus, God and the Holy Spirit. The three main branches of Christianity are Roman Catholic, Orthodox and Protestant. Within these branches there are many different denominations and expressions. These have arisen from different interpretations of the Bible and challenges to specific teachings around such things as salvation, the authority of the Bible, the sacrament, church governance and the role of leaders.

The Roman Catholic Church is the largest denomination in the world and has the Pope as its head. It was the first denomination of Christianity and was founded by Peter, one of Jesus' disciples or followers. As well as baptism, the Roman Catholic Church regards practices of confirmation, confession, marriage, holy orders and the anointing of the sick as sacraments or sacred actions. Baptism and confirmation are viewed as the entrance sacraments to the church with confession and Holy Communion as the regular necessary 'feeding' sacraments. It is the traditional Roman Catholic belief that Holy Communion is

WOMEN IN CHRISTIANITY

The Bible teaches that 'There is neither Jew nor Greek, slave nor free, male nor female, for you are all one in Christ Jesus' (Galatians 3: 28). However, across different cultures women are often still seen as unequal to men. Some Christian traditions do not permit women to lead, worship or train as religious leaders. There may be an understanding that the husband is the head of the family and this will be worked out in various ways. There is a strong feminist movement within Christianity that seeks to redress the balance of many centuries of patriarchal influence on the interpretation of the Bible and the church's teachings.

the actual body and blood of Christ transformed from bread and wine during the service of the Mass (transubstantiation).

The Orthodox Church is an umbrella term for many church traditions that draw on Greek, Middle-Eastern and Russian traditions. They are self-governing but emphasize the importance of tradition. Prayer and fasting form an important part of Orthodox Christianity. They usually follow a slightly different calendar (Julian) to Roman Catholics and Protestants, which means that festivals are celebrated on different dates. Protestantism is an umbrella term for many church traditions that include, for example, the Church of England, Methodist, Baptist, United Reform, Lutheran, Episcopalian, Pentecostal and Charismatic churches. There are many more examples. Protestantism came about in the 16th century when there was a decisive split from the Roman Catholic Church. Protestants reject the authority of the Pope and also have varying styles of worship and rituals. Within these denominations are different churches and varied interpretations of Christian teaching. Additionally, Quakers, Seventh Day Adventists, Jehovah's Witnesses and Latter Day Saints (Mormons) have their roots in Christianity.

For the purposes of simplicity, where relevant to medicine and healthcare, the views of different denominations and sects are explained.

Names and greetings

Some Christian families may name their children after significant Biblical figures, such as Adam, Elijah, Mark or Mary. Joshua is a version of Jesus, and Jesus is a popular first name in many Spanish-influenced countries. The word 'goodbye' means 'God be with you'. Some Christians may part with 'God bless you'.

Family life

Children and young people may or may not be used to Christian practices such as prayers at home, reading the Bible as a family (especially before going to bed), giving thanks (saying grace) before a meal. Children and young people may be encouraged to tell their friends about Jesus and the Christian message. Some Christians will wear a cross as a symbol of their faith, a fish symbol, or a bracelet with a Christian message on it, for example, but these are personal choices and not part of a particular Christian tradition. Some Christian children and young people will have gone to church, Sunday school, church youth groups, uniformed organizations, such as Boys' or Girls' Brigade, or a church school. Often churches are the main basis for a lot of social interaction and support.

Views on abortion are not uniform but some Christians are opposed to abortion, with specific exceptions in certain circumstances. Some Christians would have religiously informed moral dilemmas about in-vitro fertilization (IVF). There are usually strong beliefs against euthanasia and suicide due to the belief that God is the creator of life and should decide when it ends.

There are no universally prohibited substances, and no specific religious teachings about birth rites, breast-feeding, adoption and fostering, although there may be significant cultural influences. Some traditions will be against the use of contraception.

Some traditions will have teachings that affect diet, such as periods of fasting (e.g. Lent), the tradition of eating fish on Fridays and the prohibition of alcohol. However, these are not universal teachings and should not be assumed.

Languages

Christianity is a worldwide religion. Christians can speak any language and read the Bible in their own language. Although originally written in Hebrew and Greek, there is no special religious merit attributed to reading the original languages.

Stories and attitudes to children

Children learn about Christian faith from family, the church community and sometimes school. Jesus taught that children have a special place in God's kingdom. Some children will be baptized as a baby or young child. Some traditions believe that the person needs to make an informed decision to commit to the faith, and therefore would profess their faith, perhaps through a baptism, at an older age or through confirmation of their baptismal vows. Jesus is described as the Son of God and the importance of a parental relationship with God the Father may be emphasized to children. Thus, some Christians would understand themselves to be 'Children of God' or 'friend of God' – in relationship and under God's care and love. Many Christians would also understand that they are made in the image of God, including sick or disabled children. A key story about children in the Bible says:

> At that time the disciples came to Jesus and asked, 'Who, then, is the greatest in the kingdom of heaven?' He called a little child to him, and placed the child among them. And he said: 'Truly I tell you, unless you change and become like little children, you will never enter the kingdom of heaven. Therefore, whoever takes the lowly position of this child is the greatest in the kingdom of heaven. And whoever welcomes one such child in my name welcomes me.' (Matthew 18: 1–5)

Many Christians would understand that children are a gift and blessing from God and have wisdom about God.

Role models

Many Christians would understand Jesus to be the perfect role model and would try to lead their lives by following his example. Christians sometimes ask, 'What would Jesus do?' when trying to decide a moral solution for a problem or to remind them about how Jesus acted with justice and compassion. In some traditions, particularly Roman Catholic, Mary, the mother of Jesus, is a significant person. Children and young people will perhaps have been told some of the well-known Bible stories where particular characters can be seen as role models, such as Noah, Moses, Esther, Deborah, Daniel and Peter and those of the saints.

Care of Christian patients and their families in hospital

Christians differ in the details of their beliefs and practices, so the information given here should be seen as a guide from which to ask further questions. There is a wide spectrum of beliefs within the Christian faith and within these traditions a further spectrum of how seriously they take their religion, so it is very important to have a conversation with families and children without making assumptions.

Food and prohibited products

Some Christians observe Friday as a day when they do not eat meat. Some Christians may wish to fast before receiving Holy Communion and during Lent (40 days before Easter). Some abstain from alcohol. There will be very precise beliefs within some traditions, such as Jehovah's Witnesses, who do not permit blood transfusions based on their interpretation of specific Bible passages. Similarly, they do not agree with procedures that involve the removal and storage of their own blood, for example blood donation, because of the belief that blood removed from the body is unclean. There may be different opinions for autotransfusion, where the patient receives their own blood for transfusion – it is important to ask. The right of a patient to refuse a procedure on religious grounds should always be respected, as long as they are found to be mentally competent to understand the risk. Gillick Competence and Fraser Guidelines are important considerations for paediatric patients in the UK.[2]

Modesty and hygiene

There is nothing specifically relevant in healthcare to say about modesty and hygiene, and generally there are no restrictions on same-gender care from a Christian perspective. There may be many cultural considerations depending on where the child and family are from. Some Christians may be reluctant to remove jewellery depicting religious symbols, such as a crucifix on a necklace. There may be some conservative ideas about modesty, particularly in teenagers.

Members of the Latter Day Saints (Mormons) might be wearing an undergarment that covers the whole body. It is to encourage modesty and serves as a reminder of the commitment the person has made to a righteous life during a special ceremony called the Temple Endowment ceremony. This may be relevant to older teenagers who have participated in this ceremony (it is not required of children) and they may not wish to remove this garment.

Taboos

There is very little that would cause universal offence across different ages and traditions. Blaspheming (using the name of God/Jesus in vain as a swear word) is offensive to many Christians.

There may be a belief that an unbaptized child will not go to heaven, so that a family may wish for their baby or child to be baptized if there is a threat to life. This may especially apply to a family who have a Christian heritage or culture, but the importance of baptism may be a cultural concern or expectation rather than necessarily religious. In the past, unbaptized children were not usually allowed to be buried in consecrated ground, and an element of folk religion can linger around this.

Some Christians will have little understanding of the biological and social causes of mental health problems, and within some Christian communities people believe that Christians cannot or should not get depressed or anxious because of their belief in the good news of Jesus' message. The need to challenge stigma around mental health in relation to faith is a priority for many Christians.

Some Christian communities and denominations teach that homosexuality is wrong, sinful or not part of God's 'plan' for the world. Having a child or teenager who is gay in a Christian family may be a taboo, but for some may not be an issue. Some Christian traditions would also believe that sex outside of marriage was wrong and a sexually active teenager may cause problems for some families. In some circumstances the child may not want their family to be aware of some of their lifestyle choices and confidentiality is important.

By the bedside

The offer of a referral to chaplaincy will be important to some Christian children and families as a part of their hospital visit. For others it becomes important when, for example, there is a critical incident with the child, breaking bad news or a significant point of transition: such as going into life-limited, palliative, end-of-life treatment and bereavement. At these times the family and/or child may want to see a chaplain for prayer, confession, a blessing or spiritual comfort and assurance. The chaplain can then visit the family and assess what they wish. There will be no assumption on behalf of the chaplain on what is needed as there are no mandatory religious needs. The first thing the chaplain will do is to assess what is needed in the situation. There are occasions when it appears that a particular family member is urging that religious care be offered. Grandparents in particular may adopt a guardian-of-the-faith role in the family but sometimes the child is keener than the parents for religious rituals.

Baptism is a ceremony that people undertake when they decide to make a Christian commitment (or their parents decide they want to make a commitment to bring the child up as a Christian). This involves being sprinkled with or immersed in water, and can take place anywhere, anytime. Some Christian chaplains will offer this baptism or provide it on request for a child or teenager in hospital. This is particularly important to Roman Catholic families. Blessings can be offered to the child and family. These are not magic or an attempt to twist God's arm, but instead impart God's love and wisdom. However difficult the situation, such prayers and actions are offered with the assurance that 'whether we live or whether we die we are the Lord's'.

Age-specific considerations
Babies

Families with children of all ages should be offered prayers before operations, but this can be a very special and supportive intervention for babies. Some families may choose to have a naming ceremony for a baby or infant, instead of a Christening, thus permitting the child to make their own commitment to the faith when they are older.

EMERGENCY BAPTISM – A CHAPLAIN'S VIEW

Our Cathedral's priest asked me to remind parents that if we baptize their baby in the hospital that will be the official baptism. It will not be repeated later in the parish, except for a service of completion. He also asked me to remind families that the church no longer teaches that unbaptized babies go to Limbo (a place between heaven and hell). Instead, he encourages parents, if they are concerned for their baby, to make plans for baptism and know that the church teaches the 'Baptism of Intention': that if their baby were to die before that baptism is accomplished, God treats that baby as having been already baptized. This allows us to explore the fears behind the parents' request, which are often more about medical issues and very often fears greater than are justified by the baby's true condition. The priest was trying to help us avoid unnecessary 'emergency baptisms' in the hospital.

In an emergency baptism, the Catholic Church teaches that anyone can baptize. It is a matter between God and the one being baptized, so a non-Catholic (or even non-believer) may baptize. Knowing this, we offer the parents the chance to pour the water and pronounce the words of baptism. Who better? And this makes one special aspect of a baptism that in all other ways is not what they had hoped for. Not all parents are comfortable with this, of course, so we are happy to be the officiants for them. (Rev Mark Bartel, Orlando, Florida)

Children

Children may miss their home church or friends from church activities. Contact could be made for them, or they could be invited to similar groups if available in the hospital. Chapel could also be offered. Children and young people may also appreciate age-appropriate versions of the Bible and may also enjoy poetry, prayers and storybooks.

Children of all ages may enjoy craft activities that involve the Christian celebrations and are important for practising the faith (more than just cultural) such as creating an advent calendar using pictures from the Christmas story, decorating a candle or holder, or writing a prayer. A child who is a practising Christian may find comfort in holding prayer beads or a prayer cross, and such a gift can lend strength and meaning to a time of blessing or prayer.

GOOD PASTORAL CARE – A CHAPLAIN'S VIEW

As a Chaplain working in a children's hospice, I visit the children, from all faith backgrounds, who are in for respite every day; their parents and family members as well if they are present. These visits build up trust and good pastoral relationships with all. Many of the children have intellectual and sensory disabilities and complex medical conditions. Prior to visiting the children and young people, I would always ask permission from the family. To date, parents welcome my pastoral visits. The hospice ground is neutral for all of us. I often think it is the neutrality of space we share in this scenario that disarms us. I believe this disarming allows the Spirit of God to come among us in our presence, in our conversations, in our vulnerabilities to help us to connect and feel safe to engage. (Thomas Begley, lay Roman Catholic chaplain, Ireland)

Teenagers

For some committed Christian teenagers it would be important to receive Holy Communion, also called Mass or Eucharist. This would involve the church leader, priest or chaplain sharing with them bread, symbolic of Jesus' body, and either wine or grape juice, symbolic of Jesus' blood. For some Christian traditions, it is important that a young person who has made the decision and outward commitment to Christianity, through baptism, should be treated as an adult who can make informed choices about their religious faith and how to practise it. Older children and teenagers may find worship music, either traditional or contemporary, to be important. Some children who have been confirmed may wish to receive communion (Roman Catholic or Church of England) or the sacrament of the sick (Roman Catholic).

Working with the family

It may be that older members of the child's family believe in Christianity more strongly than their children and grandchildren, and may encourage more religious intervention. Pastoral support in the form of continued visits to a family, where a trusting relationship is built, are very important. There may be a sense of such feelings as guilt, and these should be taken seriously. The needs of the parents are met and supportive care is offered by a chaplain who can offer a listening ear and emotional support. The chaplain's main job may be to listen, support, encourage and befriend. Chaplains are also able to help the family explore and process some of the questions, doubts or anger they may have over their child's illness, for example. Sickness is not usually seen by Christians as punishment from God, although there are some who may express this thought.

Conducive environment

There are very few artefacts that every Christian family will want around their bed space. A Bible is likely to be the most obvious. Some will also like a cross, cards with blessings, prayers or Bible text on them, rosary beads (Roman Catholic). In some traditions, holy water is used. Space to be alone, for quiet prayer or reflection, should be available, either as curtains round the bed, quiet rooms, multifaith rooms or the chapel. Play spaces can also be an opportunity for spiritual expression.

It is important to identify religious needs early on with a family and not to offer referral to chaplaincy too late if a child is dying. For some families it is very important that their child is baptized and some chaplains will not baptize a dead child, which may cause the family further distress. Chaplains may also help facilitate discussions around organ donation, withdrawal of treatment and other aspects of end-of-life care.

Views of suffering

For many Christians, suffering is a difficult topic. Many Christians struggle with the belief that a loving God allows pain, suffering and death. This may be particularly difficult with untimely death or terrible suffering. Some Christians may see the suffering of fellow Christians as somehow unjust, particularly if they believe they are God's children or have a special relationship with God. Some Christians turn to the Biblical story of Job, a man who made an ultimate faith confession in his darkest moment. He experienced poverty, sickness and bereavement but still believed that God had a purpose for his life. Reading the Psalms in the Bible may also be of comfort as in them the whole range of emotions are expressed. Psalm 23 and Psalm 121 are particular favourites. Many Christians will also find comfort in the story of Jesus' suffering and death. The Bible tells the story of Jesus experiencing suffering, physical pain as well as crying out to God in emotional pain, and God entered the pain of our human experience in Jesus and promises to be with his followers through every experience of life. Because Christians believe that Jesus is now in heaven, he is there still bearing the scars of his crucifixion. Some Christians will understand that suffering is a universal experience of all human beings and it may be understood as a way to demonstrate empathy and shared experience. Some Christians

> ### SYMBOLS, CANDLES, LIGHT AND HEARTS
>
> Symbols speak where words sometimes don't, especially in times of loss, grief, hope or remembrance. Symbols such as light, candles, water, fabrics, essential oil, incense, forget-me-not flowers, colour, a memory tree or prayer tree, a child's toy, musical instrument or football team's scarf are used as ways of praying creatively, offering hope to a family and remembering children and teenagers who have died.

will understand pain and suffering to be God's will, the work of Satan or the Devil. For some Christians the suffering of children may cause them to question or lose their faith; for others it is a time of growing in faith. This is a particular area where there has been a fusion of religious and cultural values and therefore the principles of assessment and asking are of the utmost importance.

> ### UNDERSTANDING SUFFERING – A CHAPLAIN'S VIEW
>
> I always assure parents that what has happened to their child is not a direct judgement from God on their family, that it is not God's revenge. I will also assure them that God wishes to be with them and loves them no matter what happens. I find that the well-known poem 'Footprints' often has a lot of significance during times of suffering and I will explore this with the family. This is a poem we have found relates to people of many faiths or none.

Attitudes to medical care

Most Christians would welcome medical care. There are many references in the Bible to seeking healing through bandages and salves, as well as references to seeking help from physicians (Colossians 4: 14;

Matthew 9: 12). Some Christians believe that God works miracles and can heal through supernatural causes but also through modern medicine and scientific advances. Many Christians would understand their personal responsibility to take care of their body and mind. In some sects of Christianity, such as the Christian Science movement, there may be a teaching that seeking the help of a doctor is an indication of lack of faith in God's ability to heal – this is not a common teaching across Christianity.

Understanding illness and disease

There are no religious objections to life support. However, there may be some concerns in certain traditions that this comes close to 'playing God' and there may be some reservations on these grounds. Some sects within Christianity, such as the Latter Day Saints (Mormons) suggest that steps to prolong life longer than naturally necessary should not be taken. There may be some cultural superstitions about blood exchange, but there is no religious objection to receiving or donating blood or organs.

> **RELIGIOUS INVOLVEMENT IN DECISION-MAKING**
>
> It may be very important to seek advice from a chaplain or Christian leader if the family have religious concerns around life support, blood transfusion and refusal of medical help in favour of prayer/God's healing alone. If the family is devout, they may seek religious guidance to inform every medical decision.

Understanding mental illness

Some people with Christian beliefs would understand mental illness to be another health problem, with psychological causes. Others may believe that mental illness is a spiritual issue, perhaps caused by sin, demonic forces or lack of faith. Across all cultures and faiths there is huge stigma associated with mental illness. Some Christians will be reluctant to accept medication for mental health problems, believing instead that spiritual cures, such as prayer or in some cases exorcism, are the only solutions. Unfortunately, the general social stigma surrounding mental health problems will be reinforced if only spiritual solutions and understandings are offered to Christian families. Some Christians would understand that someone attempting suicide may not be mentally well, and this would be understood by a loving and merciful God. Because of the high regard for the sanctity of life, Roman Catholics have particular concerns around suicide.

A CHAPLAIN'S EXPERIENCE

A 15-year-old boy was being treated on the mental health ward for psychotic symptoms, and a chaplain's visit was requested. Eddie was worried about the nature of his sins and whether or not he was likely to go to hell as a result. Over a period of several weeks, the chaplain visited regularly, bringing an attitude of acceptance and encouragement offering prayers expressing God's reassurance and love and addressing some of Eddie's fears. The nurse appreciated the weekly visits, commenting that Eddie did not get many visits from home.

Pain management

Most Christians will accept medicine for pain management, although Christian Scientists do not agree with medication, instead believing in God's healing powers. Prayer is sometimes used to manage pain and suffering. There is a belief in Christianity that one can express one's burdens, worries and problems to God and God hears the person's petition for help, strength, grace and comfort.

Traditional healing and medicine

There are several Christian traditions that would emphasize miraculous healing. In some traditions, large groups may visit to offer prayers and songs with the belief that these will directly help the child's health. Directing the group to a side room may be appropriate as these prayer-healing rituals may get passionate and cause unintentional disruption on the ward.

Christianity is a worldwide religion, and can be found in every country and across all cultures. For this reason there may be strong cultural influences around health and healing that are not specifically religious or Christian but are strongly held beliefs. Some people will blend cultural traditions with the Christian message, and will practise a faith that mixes these two elements together. Their beliefs can be complex and not easily categorized into a specific Christian denomination. For example, some people will rely on herbal remedies, massage, acupuncture and dietary restrictions or changes. Some of these will have an evidence base for their efficacy and some practices will provide reassurance to the person without having much physical effect.

Understanding death

Christians believe that there is a life after death. Nevertheless, life is precious from conception until death and efforts should be made to preserve it. Pain is usually to be treated or alleviated even if, occasionally, this means that death occurs earlier than might otherwise be the case. There are a range of Christian beliefs about heaven, ranging from individuals being judged by a holy and loving God to everyone being given a chance to accept God's gift of salvation even after death. There is no clear age at which a child might be expected to take personal responsibility for their own faith and life, and it is widely believed that all babies and very young children who die are not dead but alive with Christ in heaven. In heaven, there is a community of loved ones and other Christians that the child would be going to join. It is never God's will that children should die or indeed that anyone should die before their natural span of life. Jesus also has a very special place for children in his ministry, indicating that the qualities of a child are necessary to enter into heaven or to have a special relationship with him. Such qualities include innocence, trust, the ability to love, joy and wonder.

Preparing for death

A baptism (sometimes known as a Christening) can take place. This can be done anywhere, including an operating theatre if the child might die in surgery, although this is far from ideal. In some Christian traditions, baptism can be performed after death although some Christian chaplains, priests or ministers will not wish to do this. A naming ceremony can also be offered. Family and friends can participate in reading the Bible, saying the Lord's Prayer, other prayers and Holy Communion. Touch may be used as a therapeutic comfort – for example, holding the child or touching the child's head during blessing or prayer. Death is the moment of passing from this earthly life into a heavenly one, where an all-loving God is present and all pain and suffering will be ended.

When a child is approaching death:

- Non-verbal actions can be more important as death approaches. Silence can be very respectful.

- Close family members will want to be involved as the priest/ pastor/minister says special prayers. However, large numbers from some cultures/traditions may be present.

- Even if the family have a local priest they are in contact with, it's important that they're offered chaplaincy support too.

- Practising Catholics and Orthodox Christians may want a priest for confession, Holy Communion or last rites (sacrament of the sick) at such a time. The child knows the wrongs she or he has done are forgiven by God.

- Any special toys, a crucifix or cross, and a Bible may be important to have nearby.

- The family may need space away from, as well as ties at, the bedside.

- The child may be anointed with oil as part of a final ritual and blessing.

- In general, a good death should include good pain management, the family should be kept constantly informed of what is happening, and suitable religious support and cultural rituals, such as taking footprints or handprints, should be offered.

Immediately after death:

- The eyes are closed and last offices (prayers) can be performed.

- Hygienic washing of the body can be carried out by hospital staff. It is unlikely that a religious ritual washing will be performed.

> **CONDOLENCES**
> Sympathy cards are commonly sent, and/or cards with prayers or inspirational verses. Those close to the family and neighbours are likely to visit.

- Most Christian families will welcome the offer of, for example, footprints to be taken.

- It is important to leave religious jewellery intact or to ask the family if they want it returned to them.

Organ donation and post-mortem

Sacrifice and helping others are key themes across all forms of Christianity, therefore a decision to donate organs is seen as a positive action in most Christian denominations, and Christians would express gratitude upon receiving an organ, as it would be considered a gift. However, this is still a matter of personal choice. There are no religious concerns about post-mortem. However, there may be cultural fears or concerns about what a post-mortem involves.

Hospice care

There are unlikely to be any religious objections to hospice care. However, there may be some general societal misunderstanding of what a hospice offers.

Caring for the family after the death of their child

Questions about suffering and the goodness of God are raised in an acute way at a time of great stress. Special considerations apply if it is an interfaith partnership (including where one partner is Christian and the other has no faith) for parents and siblings. There are specialist Christian counselling agencies as well as secular agencies, which are particularly useful where accepted doctrines of hope and love do not match feelings of grief and anger, for example. The offer of comfort booklets, cards and memorials are commonly appreciated.

The funeral

Families may choose burial, or cremation and then the burial of the child's ashes. There are no major religious teachings on cremation or burial. Some Christians may interpret the (future) resurrection and unification with God as literal, and therefore may not want to cremate in order to keep the body intact. There are cultural, financial and ecological considerations in deciding on the nature of a burial or cremation. Undertakers are usually involved and the family's local priest/pastor/minister. Sometimes a member of the chaplaincy team will conduct the funeral.

The service can be a time of thanksgiving for the child's life and an opportunity to remember the child in creative ways through, for example, photographs, poetry, or their favourite colour or song being included creatively in the service. Chaplains can help with child-specific resources for the service. Cemeteries and crematoria often have special areas of remembrance for babies. In the Catholic tradition, the funeral is a Mass.

Continuing bonds

There is likely to be a strong belief that the child is now in heaven and is now at peace and no longer suffering. Continuing bonds ('Is she still with me?', 'I see her in the garden') is not a traditional Christian belief, as the soul is believed to be with God in heaven. However, this notion may bring comfort and in the short term would not be discouraged by a pastoral carer. There may also be a belief in the child becoming an angel, or that guardian angels are watching over the child and/or the family. Anniversaries such as birthdays, Christmas and the anniversary of the death may be marked through visits to the grave, prayers and other special rituals. The child may be remembered by raising money for charity. Many hospitals and churches offer annual memorial services or events which families may wish to participate in. Churches often do this around All Souls Day, 2 November.

Key festivals

Epiphany: Twelve days after Christmas when the gifts of the wise men are remembered.

Shrove Tuesday: The day before Lent begins when traditionally pancakes are made and tossed.

Ash Wednesday: The beginning of Lent. Forty days of fasting and preparation for Easter.

Mothering Sunday: Halfway through Lent when the fast may be broken for one day and 'simnel cakes' are eaten. Traditionally, mothers are celebrated and visited.

Annunciation: The Annunciation celebrates the appearance of the Angel Gabriel to Mary when she was told she would be the mother of Jesus.

Maundy Thursday: The night before Good Friday when Jesus sharing the Last Supper with his disciples is commemorated.

Good Friday: The Friday before Easter commemorates the death of Jesus by crucifixion.

Easter Sunday: The day Christians celebrate the resurrection of Christ – the most important Christian festival.

Pentecost: When Christians celebrate the gift of the Holy Spirit.

Ascension: Marks the last earthly appearance of Christ after his resurrection. Forty days after Easter, Christ ascended into heaven.

Harvest: A seasonal celebration linked with gathering in the harvest and thanking God for his goodness and provision.

Advent Sunday: The beginning of the season of preparation for Christmas.

Christmas Day: The day Christians celebrate the birth of Christ.

Celebrating Christmas

Christmas is the celebration of the birth of Jesus, and often nativity plays tell the story which can be found in the Bible in the gospels of Matthew and Luke. Christmas can be celebrated by making Christmas decorations such as angels and stars, which are found in the Christmas story; making Christingles that represent Jesus as the light of the world, which are oranges with a candle, four cocktail sticks with sweets on and red ribbon round the middle (there are many guides to making Christingles online). One year, Birmingham Children's Hospital (BCH) adapted the Mexican tradition of Posada where chaplains dressed as Mary and Joseph and made a donkey, and took round nativity-themed activities for children to do.

Further reading

Beech, V. and the Paediatric Chaplaincy Network (2011) *Jesus Still Loves Joe.* Birmingham: Christian Education.

Beech, V. and the Paediatric Chaplaincy Network (2011) *Sam's Special Book.* Birmingham: Christian Education.

Nash, P. (2011) *Supporting Dying Children and their Families.* London: SPCK.

Notes

1   With thanks to Kathryn Darby for her contributions to this chapter.
2   See NSPCC, *A Child's Legal Rights: Gillick Competency and Fraser Guidelines,* at www.nspcc.org.uk/Inform/research/briefings/gillick_wda101615.html for more details.

4

CARE OF A HINDU CHILD AND FAMILY

Madeleine Parkes and Rakesh Bhatt[1]

Introduction to Hinduism

Hinduism, often referred to as the 'oldest living religion', is an umbrella term for a way of life full of spirituality and ritual that originated in India. 'Hinduism' is a term that many Hindus wouldn't recognize – the Hindu religion and spirituality are a way of life so deeply interwoven with daily life that viewing them as a belief and practice that one can pick up and put down when needed, or on certain holy days, is an unknown concept.

21ST-CENTURY HINDUISM

Hinduism Today, a global magazine about modern Hinduism, offers us a guide to 'What is Hinduism?':

- Following a vegetarian diet
- A reverence toward, and desire to protect, the environment
- Solving conflicts through nonviolent means
- Tolerance towards others
- Teaching that the whole world is one family
- The belief in *karma* as a system of divine justice
- The belief in reincarnation
- The practice of yoga and meditation
- Seeking to personally experience Divinity[2]

Hinduism is vast and its ideas are many, so any attempt to generalize beliefs and practices could cause problems with assumptions. Hindu denominations may be characterized by the different ways people worship, practise and interpret doctrine. There are many different types of Hinduism and, where practical and relevant, the differences between them will be provided. The information provided below on culture, religion and spirituality should be taken as a starting point, from where you can be made aware of some of the differences you may encounter. However, the golden rule always applies, no matter how much factual knowledge you have read – *ask, don't assume.*

Beliefs and rituals

Hinduism has no single founder: it has been developed by many saints, individuals and communities of people and their ideals. Most Hindus believe in one ultimate supreme God called *Brahman.* However, Brahman is depicted in many hundreds of forms and in many different ways, so it may appear that there are lots of different gods. Each different form or face of God represents different qualities of Brahman. Brahman is such an abstract and mysterious God it is important for Hindus to have more concrete representations of Brahman that can be comprehended. Hinduism, unlike many monotheistic religions, is not preoccupied with defining God too strictly as God is considered beyond our imagination, and encountering God can be deeply personal and subjective. Hinduism is very old and emerged through a rich history of scriptures and traditions. Most relevant are the *Vedas,* the *Upanishads,* the *Ramayana* and the *Mahabharat* (which includes the *Bhagavad Gita* or *Geeta*), which have remained unchanged for thousands of years. The most popular scripture today is the *Bhagavad Gita* due to its accessibility and its focus on daily practices of devotion.

Many Hindus aim to become as knowledgeable as they can about their way of life and to act out Hindu values and morals in daily life, although there are no strict set of rules that all Hindus must agree on – again 'Hinduism' describes a huge spectrum of different beliefs and ways of life, although many Hindus would agree that belief in God, belief in *karma* and reincarnation and the ancient scripts, the *Vedas,* form the basics of Hinduism. Other than these, many beliefs, practices and rituals will vary. Many rituals are regularly completed at home and within a family setting, although many Hindus will also visit the *mandir* (temple). Different temples may focus on different gods and goddesses to help people focus on one part of the ultimate reality, Brahman.

Concept of worship in Hinduism

Prayers can be said individually or collectively. Singing hymns or chanting mantras as well as meditation are important Hindu practices, both at home and at the temple. The *mandir* will provide classes and social activities for families and children, as well as being a place of worship. Different forms or images of the one God called Brahman can be depicted in statues and images. There may be male and female representations of God. It may seem that there are lots of different deities because of the variety of statues; however, they are all ultimately part of the same God. It is like a diamond – it is one gem but with lots of different faces or sides.

At the *mandir*, shoes are always removed before entering and there may be incense burning. People may also ring a bell to announce their presence to God. People can worship God by focusing their attention on individual images or statues to help them remember the qualities of God. An important part of *puja* (worship ceremony) includes the person passing their hands over a lighted lamp or candle and symbolically moving their hands over their heads to indicate that they are emerging from darkness into the light. Sanctified water is sometimes sprinkled on both people and images of God to symbolize purity and there will sometimes be singing or chanting. Visitors may bring flowers or food to offer to God as a token of their gratitude to God for providing what they need.

Denominations

There are four main traditions or branches of Hinduism that vary depending on which God or Goddess they predominantly worship. These are Vaishnavism, Shaivism, Smartism and Shaktism. Many Hindu temples (or *mandirs*) in the UK will not be aligned to a specific tradition and may include elements of many traditions.

Names and greetings

Some Hindus will greet each other with '*namaste*', which means 'I bow to the God in you.' This holds spiritual significance as the person is recognizing the divine life force in others, which is the same as that which resides in them. Sometimes '*namaste*' will be spelt and pronounced in different ways, such as '*namaskar*'. However, '*namaste*' is the most common. *Namaste* may be accompanied by a gentle bow, with hands held in a prayer position. Many Hindu children and young people will use *namaste* regularly, at any time of the day, and particularly to greet older adults as a sign of respect. Between friends and people of similar ages, it is more common to use 'hello' and 'how are you', although *namaste* can be used in addition as a mark of respect and to greet guests or visitors.

The naming of a newborn baby in Hinduism is often an important and spiritually significant event, and important religious rites around this are found in Hindu scriptures. The name that a person is given is a reminder of certain Hindu spiritual virtues, or because the name and the birthdate are thought to be auspicious.

The format may be: personal name – *religious name* – family name; for example, Arima *Kumari* Chopra. Generally, Hindu names can be any name that comes from the indigenous languages of India, such as Sanskrit. While Hindu names may be synonymous with Indian names, not all Indian names represent Hinduism. Indian names can also be associated with Jainism, Buddhism, Sikhism or Christianity.

Family life

For some Hindus, life begins at the time of conception, and abortion is disapproved of in traditional scriptures. There is a strong sense of family life and the importance of having children, not just for the individual but as a duty to society. Contraception is acceptable and IVF is permissible.

Very young children might be involved in family prayers and *puja* (worship) if these practices are common at home. The ages at which children are involved in Hindu practices are family specific and there is no right or wrong age to start involving children. Hinduism holds that the parents are the first teachers (gurus) to children and traditionally the spiritual, social and moral guidance of a child is in the hands of the parents.

Some families will involve children in worship and rituals from birth as part of living out a Hindu way of life rather than it being a separate activity only done on certain days. Festivals and major celebrations are celebrated in the temple with fellow devotees, although some practising Hindus will celebrate at home. Many different books are available for children to explain Hindu festivals, scriptures and beliefs, and may be found by the child's bedside. It is OK to ask them about what they are reading and what they find interesting about their religion – this is good spiritual care.

WOMEN IN FAMILY LIFE

Daily worship (*puja*) is often, but not always, performed by the mother on behalf of her family. Many Hindu homes will have the corner of a room or possibly a whole room as a dedicated *puja* space, and this space will often have a shrine to the gods and goddesses the family have chosen to worship. Women mostly take care of the religious education of the children in the family and the traditional view that women look after the home, including the children and the gods that visit the shrine, is a view that is still present in many families. Note that it is considered a duty but also an honour to be the one responsible for providing for the children and the gods.

Languages

The family may have roots in or have emigrated from India or Nepal. India has several languages, faiths and cultures. Therefore, Hindu families could have a variety of cultural traditions and differences, including language and customs associated with their faith. There are over 900 million Hindus worldwide so you can expect a huge range of cultures and languages. Some of the more common languages might include Hindi, Urdu, Punjabi and Gujarati. The ancient language Sanskrit is the language the sacred texts of Hinduism are written in. Although this language is read and spoken for religious purposes it is not commonly used in conversation.

Stories and attitudes to children

Children play a key role in the Hindu faith. Many parents will be deeply connected with their children and involved in raising them to a high moral standard in line with Hindu teachings. There is a perception that the children represent the family in the wider community and therefore parents will be keen for children to behave well and be raised in a way that is socially acceptable. From a religious perspective both genders should be seen as a gift from God and therefore should be treated as equals. However, culturally this is not always the attitude that prevails, as sometimes boys are seen as a better gift to the family than girls because of a perceived superiority in continuing the family line and providing financial stability.

Amongst some orthodox Hindus or within some Hindu cultures, childlessness is seen as unfavourable and may generate a stigma for a couple who cannot, or have not, had children. In Hindu theology the love between a mother and a child is considered the most pure, as it is believed a mother will not let her child down or intentionally mislead the child.

THE STORY OF KRISHNA AND THE BUTTER

In the popular story of Krishna stealing the butter, the god Krishna as a small child steals butter from the churn in his own house. He eventually admits to this but asks his mother if this is our house and we own everything in it, then how can I be stealing the butter? This story is used to explain to children that they should not steal even from their own family as the act of stealing in itself, no matter who it is from, is a form of lying and is morally wrong.

Overall, Hinduism emphasizes that children should be loved and in no way neglected. The first chapter of the *Bhagavad Gita* speaks of the important role of a family, including grandparents or others in an 'elder' role, in order to raise children morally and promote a good society. The son of a parent who has recently died will be expected, in some families, to perform funeral rites and ceremonies for many months after death to ensure his parent's wellbeing in the afterlife. A son may be called to do this as a teenager as he may be considered an adult with adult responsibilities at this time.

Care of Hindu patients and their families in hospital

Every Hindu will be different from another in their beliefs and practices, so the information given here should be seen as a guide from which to ask further questions. Not every Hindu family, and not every member of the same family, will follow the same rules and ideas, so the golden rule of *ask, don't assume* is paramount.

Key points include:

- Daily *puja* (worship) is part of family life and can be adapted for use in hospital.

- Vegetarianism is common and this affects the use of animal products in both food and medicine.

- A sense of *karma* (simplified as 'what goes around comes around') is a strong belief in Hinduism and is used to understand suffering.

- Hindus often see the body as holistic – mind, body and spirit.

- Coloured threads and jewellery may be significant religious symbols and should not be removed without permission.

- There are likely to be large numbers of visitors.

Food and prohibited products

Many Hindus are strict vegetarians, and 'vegetarianism' can mean different things to different people. For many Hindus, vegetarian means excluding eggs as well as all meat and fish. Some Hindus, particularly those from specific coastal regions of India and Sri Lanka, may include fish in their diet. Eating cow and ox flesh is specifically scripturally forbidden for all Hindus.

For many vegetarians it is important that cutlery used to serve meat is separate from cutlery used to serve vegetarian alternatives. The family may bring food from home for the child in hospital. A child may not be eating hospital food for reasons other than illness, such as not liking the taste of hospital food or not being used to the flavours. Hindu patients and families may observe festivals throughout the year and certain fasts, which will affect dietary needs. Children are usually exempt from fasts and certainly those who are ill are exempt. Children and families may undertake a fast to mark religious festivals or important events. Fasting is encouraged to remind us not to overindulge in food and to remove our feelings of desire for food so that space can be made in our minds for more spiritual thoughts.

Some vegetarians strongly avoid animal by-products such as gelatine, which is often found in jelly, sweets and the capsules of medication. Where possible, liquid alternatives to gelatine-containing capsules should be offered; where this is not possible it should be explained to the patient and family.

Modesty and hygiene

Care provided by staff of the same gender is preferable for teenagers and young adults in order to preserve modesty. This isn't required for children who have not reached puberty, although ideas about modesty may be strong and even young children may not want to change in front of others. Hindu children may prefer to shower under running water, which is culturally preferred to a bath.

Families and children may eat with their hands, often the right hand. There is a high regard for purity, both physically and spiritually, so washing may occur very frequently, especially before consuming food. Although alcohol is not forbidden in Hinduism it is often restricted or unused due to beliefs about physical wellbeing and spiritual purity. For this reason families may be reluctant to use alcohol-based hand gel.

Children and teenagers from immigrant families may have a mixed identity around dress and language. Traditional dress may be worn, as well as Western clothes. Any threads or beads around a child's wrist, chest or neck should be respected as religious symbols and should not be removed without consultation. Additionally, members of the family may be wearing a smudge mark or coloured dot on their forehead. This should be respected as a symbol of faith and culture, and often represents meditation and wisdom. It is commonly known as a *bindi* or *tilak*.

Taboos

Taboos and stigmas are still big problems in many Hindu communities due to the fear of speaking out. Children may also suffer as they may be forbidden to talk about certain subjects. For many Hindus, premarital sex is a significant taboo and is becoming increasingly discouraged as Western practices become more influential. Discovering a teenager or young adult has had premarital sex could cause problems in the family as they may worry about the response of the wider community. A lack of communication within families about topics regarding sex and health can be common. Concern for sexual health is not viewed as important for young people because many Hindu parents assume their children are virgins until they are married.[3] This is still considered the ideal sexual morality in traditional Hindu culture, and public signs of affection may be discouraged. Gender identity has been a fluid concept in Hinduism, with some gods changing their gender. Hindu views of homosexuality are varying and diverse, in part because the accepted Hindu religious texts do not explicitly mention homosexuality. For some Hindus there is a religious taboo around menstruation, which is believed to make the woman spiritually unclean. The woman must have a ritual bath or wash in order to participate in religious ceremonies. For other Hindus, a young woman's first menstruation is celebrated.

Hinduism recognizes that alcohol and drugs can be powerful substances; however, it does not have a blanket ban on these items. Once again, due to the diversity within Hinduism, many Hindus will have different opinions on this.

Mental illness, explored in detail below, brings its own challenges. Suicide and attempted suicide are considered forbidden by most Hindu thinkers. The view that all life is sacred is paramount, as is the understanding that the frame of mind at the moment of death has a significant influence on the next incarnation. To take one's life in despair leads to a future life of even greater despair and so the ending of one's own life in such circumstance is deemed the greatest spiritual transgression. To sacrifice one's own life selflessly and with composure and dignity is not frowned on and praised as the highest service.

By the bedside

Most children, including very young ones, will be wearing a red thread around their wrist. Sometimes this will be a string of beads, or for infants on their sixth day on earth, a delicate white thread may be tied on their wrist or neck. This is a tangible symbol of blessing; they may have been on a pilgrimage in India or have been blessed by a local priest. The thread cannot be removed until it wears away and falls off naturally, as the blessing is carried by the thread and it would no longer be effective if the thread is broken. Parents and wider family members may also be wearing threads on their wrists. Holy books (usually the *Bhagavad Gita*) may be kept near their bed. It is popular for practising Hindus to have a *murti* or picture of god(s) in visible sight of them. These items will be brought from home by the family. Do not touch or remove any religious or cultural objects from the room or the child without asking permission to do so.

Many Hindus will pray differently, or to different gods, and there are no set rules as to when and where they should pray. Some families may wish to know where the multifaith or prayer room is; others may draw the curtains and pray by the child's bedside.

'Devout Hindu women may believe their vows and fasts will protect their husband and children.'[4] This is particularly relevant when the child is in hospital as the mother and perhaps other family members may wish to offer prayers and fasts in the belief that this may help their child recover.

Although the child, siblings and perhaps parents will speak and understand English, it is likely that older generations will not. Even parents who have a good level of English may find medical terminology difficult to understand, as they may not have heard it before and the concepts may not be easily translatable.

A translator may be needed; the likely languages spoken by Hindus include Hindi, Punjabi, Gujurati, Urdu, Tamil and Bengali. However, there are many additional languages spoken in India where many Hindus are from, and increasingly Hindus are living in parts of Africa, the Middle East and East Asia so there could be a variety of languages spoken.

Every effort should be made to use a professional translator, not a family member of the patient. Where practicable, a chaplain may be able to offer translation skills. If using a family member to translate, be very mindful that they are hearing the news you are telling them for the first time and may not fully understand what is being said. If they do understand they may not be able to find the most accurate words to translate the information into – this is particularly true for unfamiliar medical terminology or concepts – and they should be invited to clarify their understanding with you.

Note that Hindu holy scriptures were originally written in Sanskrit, which is an ancient language no longer in conversational use today. However, it may still be spoken when reading holy scriptures.

A CHAPLAIN'S VIEW

My first duty as a priest and chaplain, rather than speaking, is just to come and be with the child. Families and patients are fond of a familiar face, and it brings relief that somebody is present, walking with them on a difficult journey.

My role is to support, whilst being non-judgemental, anything from a few minutes up to an hour, and I'm always led by the family. I regularly visited a 16-year-old boy and his family who were shocked with his diagnosis of a terminal illness. I walked the whole journey with them, through treatments, palliative care and death, and witnessed without prescribing or judging the child and family's journey.

I offer universal prayers of comfort but never say, 'I will visit you next week' as I don't know what will happen before then.

Age-specific considerations
Babies

Many Hindu babies will go through a naming ceremony, called *namakarana samskara*. This usually happens within a month of their birth, and during this ceremony the baby and their name is presented to God for blessings, and the baby is welcomed into the Hindu religion. This ceremony can take place at a local temple or in the home, with the presence of a Hindu priest and the family. After the sixth day, a baby may have a delicate white thread tied on to their wrist or neck. This is a symbol of blessing and should not be cut or removed. It is customary in some Hindu families for the umbilical cord to be buried on the sixth day after birth.

Milk from cows is usually accepted to feed babies. Allow mothers to breast-feed, and a baby bank is allowed if needed. Some mothers may delay breast-feeding for a period of a few days, preferring to feed newborn babies with honey and sugar water. This practice has ancient religious roots and is common practice today, although families may not be aware that honey may contain botulism spores that can lead to botulism poisoning, especially for infants under 12 months.

Infants

When weaning infants on to solid food, consider if they should be fed vegetarian food, and with what restrictions, according to family wishes. Be aware of any white or red threads tied around the infant's wrist, neck or chest, and do not remove them without permission.

Children

Children and teenagers may have red threads tied around their chest, neck or wrist. These should not be removed without permission. Children and teenagers may be involved in temple (*mandir*) and community life, so ensure that they know about the availability of the multifaith room and chaplaincy/spiritual care services.

Teenagers

Teenagers are considered adults from a religious perspective when they reach puberty, although this may not be reflective of their emotional maturity. This has implications for their role in religious family life, such as presiding at funeral ceremonies. Children and teenagers have a responsibility to their parents to respect them and look after them. If a parent dies, the oldest son, even if he is still a child, bears a large amount of the responsibility for ensuring the parent is spiritually cared for.

Provide same-gender care for teenagers and young adults to preserve modesty. Another family member may wish to be present if same-gender care cannot be provided for examinations.

Working with the family

Grandparents often, though not always, live with the parents and child. It is not uncommon for extended family or many generations to live as one family unit, due to Hinduism's emphasis on strong family life. For this reason, medical staff should seek to involve grandparents and other key family members, as identified by the parents, in medical decision-making.

Similarly, the wider family, where possible and when agreed by the parents, should be kept informed as much as possible. This is essential in order to ensure the correct religious and moral decisions can be made in the best interests of the child, but without causing offence or misunderstanding. For example, consult with the family, alongside the Hindu chaplain, beforehand if the sacred red thread present on a child's wrist has to be removed before going into theatre.

Research into cultural variations on attachment theory has demonstrated that many children with roots in India have a strong attachment to the father figure.[5] This is an important consideration when working with families.

Conducive environment

There will probably be lots of family and friends wanting to see the patient, to show them that they care and want to help. Try to understand that restricting them will hurt them. Try to facilitate this where and when possible. The Hindu chaplain may be able to help, and take visitors to a free room for prayers instead of taking up space on the ward. Hindus respect the fact that a hospital ward has a medical purpose and will seek to find an alternative room for prayer and worship.

Religious items, including images of the gods and goddesses, are revered and should be treated with utmost respect. The floor and the feet can be considered spiritually impure for many Hindus, and they would not appreciate religious items being placed on the floor. Additionally, it is considered rude to make physical contact with others with feet or shoes, as this could be interpreted as insulting. However, to show respect and humility many Hindus will touch or bow at the feet of statues of the gods and goddesses.

Views of suffering

The concept of *karma* is central to understanding why there is suffering in the world for Hindus. Karmic law says that when someone does something bad it has a bad effect on their lives. Similarly, when they do something good, they can expect something good to happen in return. The effect of their actions may not be seen immediately or even in this lifetime. Therefore, when a child becomes ill it may be because they did some bad deeds in their previous lives and the results of this are being seen in this life. Blame is not placed on the child; rather, *karma* encourages people to take personal responsibility for their actions. There is no such thing as 'evil' or 'bad people', just bad actions. Ultimately, the goal of life is to escape the cycle of endless physical lives on earth by building up good *karma* and achieving oneness with God.

Regarding life after death, there is a widespread belief in reincarnation, and where the soul goes after death in this life is largely, or wholly, determined by the principles of *karma*. There is a belief that the next life is another opportunity to redress the karmic balance. For some Hindus, *karma* does not completely explain suffering. There may be a belief that suffering is the will or action of God for a greater purpose. God's purpose is ultimately a mystery. Finally, there is a cosmological understanding that the earth goes through cycles of creation and destruction, and suffering is a result of the cycle of destruction.

PARENTAL GUILT – A CHAPLAIN'S EXPERIENCE

One mum I worked with felt incredible amounts of guilt that her child had knocked a cup of hot tea over onto himself and sustained serious burns. She had a list of things that she should have done to prevent this, even though it was an accident. As a chaplain I encouraged her to move on from talking about mistakes or things she didn't do, but to admit that these actions were not done on purpose – her love for her child was being demonstrated by the permanent position she had by his bedside. Love overrides other actions and emotions. This brought her some comfort. We prayed for God's support and mercy, diverting her mind and giving her emotions up to God.

Attitudes to medical care

All medication and treatment that can provide some hope of recovery is encouraged in Hinduism. Doctors are respected and there are Hindu teachings about having the wisdom to accept the help that is being offered.

There is likely to be great appreciation of the healthcare offered to a Hindu child and family. India has no free treatment, and Western medicine offers many cures and an increased chance of survival that some Hindu families couldn't imagine if they were living elsewhere. Thanks to God would be given for the attentiveness and wisdom of staff, from consultants to cleaners, for treating them with dignity. They will appreciate anything that makes their child's illness more bearable and the child more comfortable.

As with any family with a child in hospital, it is most important to be honest with them about the current situation and the prognosis; false hope should never be given, even if it seems kinder, as the family will appreciate knowing the reality that they have to face. This is particularly true for religious families as key rituals and decisions around alleviating suffering, and around dying, will have important religious aspects that cannot be carried out without accurate and honest information. For families that have close relatives abroad it will be important to be realistic about the child's prognosis so that travel arrangements can be made for family members who wish to see the child. If you do not know an answer or are unable to give one for whatever reason, explain so honestly and offer to find out.

Understanding illness and disease

Some families will have no knowledge of some illnesses, as the illness is not known in their community, or there is lack of education around it. For example, some families don't know that small children can get cancer. This may be true for the wider family, including grandparents. There may also be a belief that if an illness hasn't been present in generations it shouldn't or can't happen to a child.

Common questions are, 'Why is this happening to us?' or 'Why me?' We can all acknowledge that this is an extremely difficult question to answer, and families and patients may look towards their religious and spiritual understanding of illness and suffering to explain this. A Hindu family may be encouraged by the chaplain to think about the present and future, focusing on caring and providing comfort for the child. Family members may want to explain suffering through their belief in *karma*, or the consequences of their actions in the past. It is written in the *Bhagavad Gita* that, 'In proportion to the extent of one's religious or irreligious actions in this life, one must enjoy or suffer the corresponding reactions of his *karma* in the next' (6:1:45). This suggests that pain is indeed the consequence of *karma*, either from this life or the past. However, one must be careful not to blame *karma* as such, but to take responsibility for one's actions. It is very difficult to understand why a child would have to suffer when he or she is technically so innocent. However, there may have been debts upon the soul inside the child that need to be cleared. The chaplain and other professionals can redirect the family's focus to the knowledge that help is available throughout this time of pain and distress, and in some cases that the illness is curable, or at least treatable.

Understanding mental illness

Many may understand mental illness to be the result of an unstable or unbalanced mind. Hindus talk about the connectedness between body, mind and spirit, and the importance of ensuring all of these are healthy and balanced. There may be a belief in the need to control the mind through thinking about positive and godly things to help improve mental health. It is known that awareness and understanding about mental illness in Asian communities is low and that stigma is high.

Mental health is a controversial issue as many Indian parents find it difficult to notice signs of mental ill health and there is a stigma surrounding the idea of seeking medical help for it. Many parents may end up scolding the children for being 'rude' or 'secluded' without realizing that the child may be showing symptoms of depression for example. They may also think that this is just 'teenage behaviour'. A family may try to conceal their son/daughter's mental illness because of the fear of the shame it will bring on the family, and the fear that their child may never marry or have a family of their own because of this shame. There may also be a

A CHAPLAIN'S EXPERIENCE

A teenage boy from a Hindu family had been admitted to hospital because of his suicide attempt. The family felt great shame and the young man wasn't communicating with them about what had happened. I talked to them both, separately, about the realities of mental illness, and the importance of finding out what happened. It was important to educate the family that the young man could be helped, medication could treat mental illness just like physical illness, and that his difficult feelings wouldn't last forever – this was to reduce the shame they felt, and the lack of knowledge they had. They needed practical information as well as cultural and religious guidance on why this happens and what to do to help.

fear that siblings are more at risk of mental illness, and that the family will only be known as 'mad'.

Lack of awareness regarding mental health means that it is often shunned in Indian communities, not spoken about, and often there is an air of embarrassment should it be revealed that the child has a mental health problem. Some Hindu priests and chaplains may increase awareness in their local communities through activities in the *mandir* (temple) and community events. There is not always adequate signposting to mental health services in these communities, and language barriers may be a problem.

Pain management

Many religious people believe, with varying degrees of strength, that pain is relieved by praying. Therefore, patients and family may conduct chants and prayers by the hospital bed. During prayer times the curtain will be drawn around the bed and the family may remove their shoes. Prayers should not be disturbed and every effort should be made to accommodate large numbers of family during this time. The *Bhagavad Gita*, a holy scripture, may be read – this holy book should not be placed on the floor, or have other items put on top of it. Prayer beads may be used and chanting may be loud. If possible, it may be appropriate to show the family, and move the patient, into a side room or direct them to another appropriate room.

Traditional healing and medicine

Ayurveda is a centuries-old philosophy of health and wellbeing that incorporates the physical, mental and spiritual. It understands optimum health to be a balance of these three energetic components of a person, and it utilizes herbal remedies to ensure this is kept so. *Ayurveda* is not regulated but is widely practised in different forms and is considered a complementary or alternative medical system just like acupuncture. It is widely respected as wise and scientific in non-Western cultures. *Ayurveda* is common in the UK as it has no known side effects. It is used mainly alongside modern treatments but not usually solely as it takes a long time to show effects. Oil for the growth of hair and honey for coughs are just two examples of simple Ayurvedic remedies which can be used instead of modern remedies. Ayurvedic remedies work so well because they do not counteract modern treatments, but work alongside them to help heal the patient faster.

The word '*Ayurveda*' literally translates as 'the science or knowledge of life'. It has roots in classical Indian texts, written in Sanskrit, and for this reason has been practised in one form or another for many hundreds, if not thousands, of years. Hindu families may use traditional home remedies. This healing system requires people to make changes to all aspects of life in order to recover from and prevent illness. *Ayurveda* is also practised on children as it is considered safe to use and part of cultural healing.

Holy ash, or *vibuthi*, may be used in different ways for different Hindus. There is a cultural belief that it cures some spiritual ailments and can have an effect on the person's physical, mental and spiritual energies. Some people use holy ash as a defence against ghosts, demons or negative energies.

Although not supported by orthodox Hindu thinking, explanations of witchcraft, the evil eye and spirit possession are perceived as the most common 'spiritual illnesses' in many Hindu families and may be seen as the cause of mental illness. As Hindus see the person holistically without separating the mind, body and spirit, it is understandable that some people see these spiritual illnesses as a cause of mental illness. This view can be both respected and explored in light of Western medicine by a chaplain.

Understanding death

Hindus believe that the soul is eternal and it encounters endless life cycles; thus it is different from the physical body and separate from it at death. Each life, good or bad, is accounted for by *karma* (the idea that 'what goes round, comes round'). Good deeds done in this life will result in a good next life. Everyone must experience the consequences of their actions sooner or later but it's possible that a person may not be able to do so in one life so they reincarnate to bear them in the next. It is recognized that

DEATH AND REINCARNATION

Nature, like living creatures, is subject to decay and destruction. But in Hindu thought there is no ultimate destruction or dissolution. It is a continuous cycle of creation, dissolution and re-creation from the dissolved state.[6]

dying is definitely painful but inevitable, for whatever is born is sure to die, and whatever dies is sure to be reborn. As the *Bhagavad Gita* (2:22) teaches, 'As a person puts on new garments, giving up old ones, the soul similarly accepts new material bodies, giving up the old and useless ones.' Children are gifts from God and He will always remember that the innocent suffered. All are rewarded accordingly. The soul is eternal and feels no pain and cannot be destroyed.

Preparing for death

In Hinduism a 'good' death is one that is at home, at an old age, painless and peaceful, where the last words spoken are the name of God. Despite the strong family connections encouraged in Hinduism, parents' decisions not to tell their child or the child's siblings bad news should be understood and treated with respect.

For children dying in hospital, life support can be used if there is a hope of recovery, but Hindu families will wish to be consulted about life support as this has religious implications. A religious leader or chaplain should be consulted.

Ideally, a child should be taken home to die with family and friends around. If this is at all practicable it would be greatly preferred and appreciated by most families. Many customs and traditions around death have been influenced by previous generations of the family, and parents/carers may turn to older family members for guidance at this time. If there are no elders present it could be important to bring in the chaplain or local religious leader to guide the family through this difficult time.

WHEN RELIGIOUS CARE DOESN'T GO WELL...

A trainee chaplain, in speaking to a family with a sick child, assured them that 'prayers do work' and offered them prayer. However, the family had received so many prayers but they were *not* working – their child was getting progressively sicker and sicker. Sometimes these well-meaning intentions can create awkwardness or difficulty. Many religious people believe that prayer is a powerful tool; however, when patients come into hospital they have already said and received lots of prayers but the child is still ill or terminally ill. It is crucial to give thought to what is said and it is important to know the context and history of the patient. Words in prayer change depending on the situation of the patient.

When a child is approaching death:

- A quiet and peaceful environment should be created (as far as this is possible).

- The family should be kept closely informed as religious practices need to be completed.

- The family should be allowed to be present and close to the child.

- The *Bhagavad Gita* or other books may be read.

- The family may wish to chant and say prayers as this is believed to relieve pain; space and time should be given for this.

- Hymns may be sung.

- There are different prayers for a dying child than for a dying adult, and the chaplain will be aware of these and can guide the family through them if required.

- There may be a request for the patient to be placed on the floor as they come close to death, in order to be closer to Mother Earth and to permit the breathing to be relaxed.

- It is customary to place holy water and tulsi leaves on the tongue of the person the moment before, or very shortly after, death so the family and chaplain should be kept informed of progress towards death.

Immediately after death:

- The eyes are closed and the last offices can be performed.

- Hygienic washing of the body can be carried out by hospital staff; however, a religious ritual wash will also be performed.

- It is preferable for a staff member of the same gender to treat the body after death.

- It is important to leave jewellery and any threads intact as these have religious significance. Additionally, do not wash off any ash or coloured markings on the forehead.

- The body should be covered with a plain cloth.

CONDOLENCES

The Hindu community are an enormous support. Individuals within the community will pass on condolences through phone calls or visits, and they may provide practical support such as cooking meals. Sending cards is not particularly common but would not be unwelcome. Hindus believe that the soul never dies; however, it may still be difficult to hear that a child has died.

Many traditional Hindus try to avoid talking about death because of the idea that bad thoughts contribute to bad things happening. There may also be some superstitious ideas about black magic as a cause of suffering or ill fortune. However, some Hindus will openly talk about death and not see it as a taboo subject.

Organ donation and post-mortem

Organ and tissue donation is permitted by many Hindu traditions as it is believed to be very good *karma*. Some families will worry about accepting organs from a deceased individual because of a belief that the *karma* of the deceased can pass to the recipient.

Hospice care

'Hospice' is not a word that easily translates into some Hindu languages, and our Hindu chaplain at the time of writing had not come across a family requesting that their child go to a hospice. There is a cultural belief amongst some Hindus that hospices are places where people die immediately and that there are strict restrictions on visiting times. There is often a lack of understanding that hospices can provide the best expertise around palliative care. Culturally, Hindus expect children and other family members to be cared for at home until death; it is seen as a parental duty to look after children at all times. There is also a belief that the 'best' death one can have is at home in peace surrounded by family, which may mean that Hindu families would not consider hospice care.

Caring for the family after the death of their child

Parents will feel helpless and in despair and most often they just need to be listened to. Do not say things like, 'I understand your pain' but try to be empathic and listen to their grief. There is no concept of continuing bonds – for example, that the child is still around looking over people as it is believed they have been reincarnated. Culturally, when someone dies – either a child or adult – members of the local community will provide the family with food for a couple of days, and visit every day for several hours to offer emotional and practical support. There are likely to be lots of visitors. Faith leaders will also visit and offer practical support in terms of the funeral. The local temple (*mandir*) is always open for prayers. Prayers, mantras and rituals will be conducted by the priest at a funeral service, which is often taken at home, although prayers will be said in the local *mandir* and the cremation will follow.

A significant difference between adults and children in Hinduism is that infants under the age of five will be buried but children over the age of five and adults will be cremated. There may be some variation about the age at which a child is buried or cremated in different traditions, as the decision is made based on beliefs about when a child begins to accrue *karma*.

The funeral

Ritual washing of the body is a religious practice and is carried out by close family members. The family will often have elders who will guide them with the most appropriate way of washing according to their tradition/denomination. New clothes will be put on and often the body will be covered in white cloth. The body may be taken home or taken away by a funeral director depending on what the family and religious leader decide. The funeral will be arranged very quickly after death where practicable, so the body should be released rapidly. Due to time pressures on the fast cremation of the body and the small number of Hindus in the community, some Hindu families may face challenges around finding a Hindu priest to conduct the funeral and finding a space at the crematorium in the time frame.

Continuing bonds

Bonds will stay through memories and remembrance. In a ritual called *punya tithi*, every year on the anniversary of the death, family and friends come together to remember and offer respects to the deceased.

Key festivals

Holi: A festival celebrating the start of spring, celebrated by throwing coloured powder and water at each other.

Mahasivrati: A festival dedicated to *Shiva*, one of the main Hindu deities.

Shri Rama Navami: The birthday of Lord Rama, an incarnation of Vishnu and the hero of Ramayana.

Raksha Bandhan: Celebrates brotherhood and love. Raksha Bandhan means 'thread of protection'.

Janamashtami: Marks the birth of Krishna, one of the most popular Gods in Hinduism – marked by singing, dancing and feasting.

Navarati: Means 'nine nights' and symbolizes the triumph of good over evil and the start of autumn.

Diwali: Festival of lights, the most popular Hindu/Sikh festival.

Celebrating Raksha Bandhan and Diwali

Raksha Bandhan, sometimes known as Rakhi, celebrates family life and love. Traditionally, sisters tie woven bracelets, rakhis, often made of red and gold thread, onto the wrists of their brothers as a symbol of gratitude. In receiving these, brothers acknowledge their responsibility to protect their sisters. Making friendship bracelets using threads, ribbons or loom bands is an activity that most can participate in as well as making rachis and exploring the idea of protection and love.[7]

Diwali is a Hindu festival also celebrated by Sikhs and Jains and is a festival of lights. It celebrates the victory of good over evil, light over darkness and knowledge over ignorance, with regional differences in the stories and legends associated with this. Small earthenware oil lamps called *diyas* are to be found in many places, and traditionally they are lit to help the goddess Lakshmi find her way into people's homes. Fireworks, including sparklers, and sweets are commonly used in Diwali celebrations. *Diyas* are made from air-drying clay and then decorated and lit using tea lights or battery-powered tea lights rather than oil for safety.

Further reading

Ganeri, A. (2008) *Stories from Faiths: Krishna Steals the Butter and Other Stories* (Hinduism). London: QED Publishers.

Zucker, J. (2005) *Lighting a Lamp: A Divali Story.* London: Frances Lincoln.

Notes

1   With thanks to Satish K. Sharma for his contribution to this chapter.

2   Quoted with kind permission from *Hinduism Today*: 'Raising Children as Good Hindus' in *What Is Hinduism?* Available at www.hinduismtoday.com/pdf_downloads/what_is_hinduism/Sec5/WIH_Sec5_Chapter37.pdf, accessed on 22 November 2014.

3   Jayaram, V. (2011) *Hinduism and Premarital Relationships.* Available at www.hinduwebsite.com/hinduism/h_premarital.asp, accessed on 20 June 2013.

4   Surgirtharajah, S. (2000) 'Women in Hinduism.' In P. Bowen (ed.) *Themes and Issues in Hinduism.* London: Continuum, p.63.

5   Pearson, J. and Child, J. (2007) 'A cross-cultural comparison of parental and peer attachment styles among adult children from the United States, Puerto Rico, and India.' *Journal of Intercultural Communication Research 36*, 1, 15–32.

6   Choudhury, A.R. (1998) 'Attitudes to Nature.' In P. Bowen (ed.) *Themes and Issues in Hinduism.* London: Cassell, p.90.

7   See Raksha Bandhan at www.raksha-bandhan.com for more information about how to make a rakhi.

5

CARE OF A JEWISH CHILD AND FAMILY

Madeleine Parkes, Rabbi Naomi Kalish and Rabbi Meir Salasnik

Introduction to Judaism

Judaism originated over 3500 years ago, and pre-dates Christianity and Islam, although these later two faiths share a history with Judaism and are collectively known as the Abrahamic traditions. Moses and Abraham are two key figures in Judaism, and the stories of their lives are very significant for Jews. Key events in the faith include the Exodus from Egypt and receiving the *Torah* on Mount Sinai. Jews will often write 'G-d' instead of 'God' out of respect for the holiness of the name and this will be done throughout this chapter. Jews believe in one G-d, who is the creator. Jews believe in having a personal relationship with G-d and in living a holy life as part of an agreement with G-d.

21ST-CENTURY JUDAISM

Today, we have an opportunity to go out and be a blessing to those regardless of their faith; that means looking outward as well as inward. I don't think we've ever had greater opportunity to express our Jewishness and share it with others. If we don't rise to that challenge, it will be our fault and we cannot blame God or the world for that.

When you talk to people, you try to show them how beautiful the world is, how complex society is and just how much of a difference each of us can make. That's my fundamental message – one of encouragement and empowerment. Let's go out there and make a difference, not just in the Jewish world, but everywhere.[1]

Jewish community and identity

When a Jew self-identifies as Jewish, that person may be referring to a religious identity like Christian or Muslim or to a cultural or ethnic identity like Irish or Italian. Twentieth-century rabbi and theologian Mordecai Kaplan asserted that Jewish identity manifests itself in three ways: belonging, behaving and believing.[2] Belonging refers to a sense of peoplehood and community. Behaving often involves observing *Halachah* (Jewish law), rituals and social activism. Believing refers to the beliefs a Jew may hold and also implies an engagement with the intellect and engagement with study. A spiritual assessment framework can be used to answer questions about these three dimensions of religious identity.[3]

Religiously, Judaism has different movements which reflect different understandings of revelation at Sinai and subsequently articulate different relationships with and practice of *Halachah*. These various branches fall broadly into two different movements: Orthodox Judaism and Progressive Judaism. Progressive Judaism includes the Liberal, Reform, Conservative and Reconstructionist movements. Orthodox Jews believe that *Halachah* is divinely given and binding; the Reform and Liberal movements place authority in the individual person to choose from Jewish law and custom what is meaningful to him or her; the Conservative Movement believes that *Halachah* is binding and historically evolving; and the Reconstructionist Movement places authority for Halachic decision-making into the hands of the community. These differences will impact the religious needs and practices of families in the hospital as well as how they make medical decisions. Culturally, Jewish identity and customs also reflect ethnic background.

The information provided below on culture, religion and spirituality should be taken as a starting point, from where you can be made aware of some of the differences you may encounter. However, the golden rule always applies, no matter how much factual knowledge you have read – *ask, don't assume.*

Beliefs and rituals

The primary sacred texts in Judaism are the Torah and the Talmud. The Torah contains the Five Books of Moses and is read during religious services from a scroll of parchment; it can also be studied in book form.

It contains 613 commandments, including the Ten Commandments. The Talmud is a written record of oral commentary and discussion on the laws and teachings of Judaism. Other sacred texts include the Prophets and the Readings in the Hebrew Bible (what constitute the Old Testament for Christians).

A Jewish child can be a bar mitzvah (boy, age 13) or a bat mitzvah (girl, age 12), which is a special coming-of-age ritual. The child from this point accepts the Jewish faith and way of life and has all the religious responsibilities of an adult Jew.

There are prayers three times a day: in the morning, afternoon and evening. Adult men (including boys over the age of 13) may wish to pray three times a day. This is likely to apply to Orthodox rather than Progressive Jews. Sometimes this happens in groups of ten as collective prayer is an important Jewish practice. The Sabbath and other special days have extra prayers in the same routine of morning, afternoon and evening. A prayer shawl (*tallit*) may be used during prayer times. Some will wear the *kippah* (skullcap) for prayer only, whereas others will wear it all the time. There is a story in the Talmud that is often told when someone is asked to summarize the essence of Judaism. During the first century BCE (before the common era) a great rabbi named Hillel was asked to sum up Judaism. He replied, 'Certainly! What is hateful to you, do not do to your neighbour. That is the Torah. The rest is commentary, now go and study' (Talmud Shabbat 31A). Hence, at its core Judaism is concerned with the wellbeing of humanity. The particulars of every Jew's individual belief system is the commentary.

Concept of worship in Judaism

Jews worship in synagogues, which may be referred to as a *shul* or temple, depending on preference. The synagogue is a place of learning and community as well as a place of prayer. Probably the most important feature of the sanctuary is the Ark, a cabinet or recess in the wall that holds the Torah scrolls. In Orthodox synagogues, men and women sit separately during religious services, sometimes separated by a balcony and sometimes by a *mechitzah,* a partition.

Judaism is a monotheistic religion. Jews believe in one G-d, who is all knowing and all present. Jews believe that G-d appointed the Jewish people to set an example of holiness and ethical behaviour to the world. Jews have a personal relationship with G-d, who continues to work in the world. Jewish faith most often takes the form of discussion of theological and existential questions, very much in the style of dialogue and exploration of the rabbis in the Talmud.

Names and greetings

In Orthodox Jewish families boys are given their Hebrew names at circumcision and girls when their fathers are called to the reading of the Torah. The traditional form of a Hebrew name for a male is [child's name] *ben* [father's name]. For a female, the form is [child's name] *bat* [father's name]. When reciting a prayer for a person's recovery from ill health, the Hebrew name will be recited as [ill person's name] *ben* or *bat* [mother's name].

Family life

Jewish law and tradition attach particular importance to the family in society and to family relationships. Both parents are responsible for the physical, emotional and spiritual nurture of children. For many families, it is important that both the mother and father are practising Jews in order to raise children in the faith. Many Jewish families prioritize their child's education.

The Sabbath, or Shabbat, is a day of rest in Jewish households that is usually of fundamental importance to family life. It traditionally begins at sundown on Friday evening and is held until sundown on Saturday evening. Many Jewish families will observe the rule of 'resting' on this day, and will not undertake any activities that could be considered work, such as cooking, cleaning, driving or lifting. For some Jewish families, switching on a light breaks this rule. It is important to recognize the significance of the Sabbath in Jewish family life, and there are very few occasions where many Jewish families would break the Sabbath – the exception would be if a child or family member is extremely unwell and needs medical attention.

Marriage is seen as an important building block of the family and is encouraged. The Progressive Jewish movements have campaigned for gay rights and same-sex marriage, although there will be many Jews who disagree with homosexual acts based on their interpretation of the Torah.

WOMEN IN FAMILY LIFE

As G-d is genderless, neither male nor female, there is no favouritism of a particular gender. Traditionally there is a belief that women and men are different. It is said that men and woman are like the brain and the heart in the physical body: both are equally vital, though each has entirely different functions, and only the normal functioning of both together ensure a healthy body, although some Jews would reject this view. Many Orthodox Jews emphasize the importance of the woman to have the main role in the house, and to be a mother and wife, which is highly respected. Recently more Jewish women have been encouraged to pursue higher education, a career and to become rabbis.

Languages

Many Jews will speak English; they may also speak Hebrew or Yiddish. Whilst many of the world's Jews live in Israel and the USA, others live in Europe and smaller numbers in South America. Therefore, a number of languages may be spoken, depending on where in the world the family are from.

Stories and attitudes to children

From a religious point of view, a child reaches the age of obligation, which means they have the same religious obligations of following laws and prayers as an adult, at 12 for girls and 13 for boys. Girls are believed to mature faster both religiously and intellectually. However, a child will often practise Judaism as an adult would, in keeping with the religious education of that child. The *Talmud* states that 'childhood is a garland of roses' and that 'the very breath of children is free of sin.'[4] Judaism recognizes that parents have the ultimate responsibility for their children, and that children will look up to their parents for guidance. Proverbs 1.8 states, 'Listen my child to the instruction of your father, and forsake not the teachings of your mother.'

Care of Jewish patients and their families in hospital

The golden rule of *ask, don't assume* is paramount. Key points include:

- Medical decisions should include the advice of a rabbi if the family are Orthodox or have traditional viewpoints.

- Many Jews will prefer to pray in a place where there are no images depicting humans or animals.

- Jewish boys will have been circumcized on the eighth day after birth.

- There are specific laws around food to be followed.

- Jewish children over the age of 12 or 13 may have the same religious obligations as an adult.

- Sabbath, from dusk on Friday to dusk on Saturday, is an important weekly time for families.

Food and prohibited products

Kosher food should be provided, which has to be sourced and prepared as *kosher*, and sealed. There are strict rules around *kosher* food, including which foods cannot be eaten. Milk and meat should not be combined – for example, a cheeseburger is forbidden. The list of laws is quite extensive. However, the most important points to consider are that Jews do not eat pork and food can only be prepared in a *kosher* kitchen. In hospitals, *kosher* meals are usually pre-packaged and can be heated in a normal kitchen if they are packaged and sealed appropriately. As many hospitals bring in frozen *kosher* meals produced by a *kosher* food company, it is important that the *kosher* symbol is identified on the packaging. It is important to provide Jewish patients with disposable plastic cutlery.

There may be some concern about medical products derived from non-*kosher* animals, for example heparin, insulin and heart valves. Where these are not received orally, there is no problem. Where the animal-based product is taken orally, if there is a non-animal based product that is as effective, that is to be preferred. Where the animal-based product provides the most effective treatment, then depending on the specific situation, it might be permitted and even obligatory to take it.

A special diet during the festival of Passover requires Jews not to eat leavened bread and cake, and in some Jewish families, rice, corn and beans are also not consumed. A special Passover meal must be provided; check with the family about their individual requirements. Matzah, unleavened bread, is a Passover replacement for bread.

Modesty and hygiene

From about the age of nine years, same-gender care may be preferable at times, such as when bathing. Sensitivity to same-gender care is appreciated. Ensure you tell the family if same-gender care is not available, particularly if the child is over the age of 12 (girl) or 13 (boy), when they are considered adult in religious terms. It may also be wise to refer the issue to the appropriate member of senior management if the family communicate dissatisfaction with the arrangements. For more Orthodox Jewish families, same-gender care could be very important. Males should be covered from belly to knees and females require a modest high neckline, and clothes that cover elbow and knees. Some Orthodox Jews do not shake hands with members of the opposite sex, and prefer only to greet them verbally.

Two pieces of religious clothing are the *kippah* (small head covering or skullcap) and *tzitzit* (a four-cornered garment with fringes at each corner) should be kept on at all times, where possible.

For teenage girls who are menstruating, traditional Jewish law states that she is spiritually 'unclean' because of the connection of menstrual blood with death. At this point she cannot participate in religious rituals and may have to have a ritual bath (*mikvah*) depending on the denomination of the family.

Taboos

The nature and extent of taboo topics in Judaism depend significantly on the denomination of Judaism adhered to and the country and culture surrounding the Jewish family.

As explained, there are Jewish laws that render certain foods 'taboo' or forbidden, and modesty rules are important. When it comes to the 'elephant in the room', some Jewish families may be shocked or challenged by issues around sexuality, pre-marital sex and pregnancy outside of marriage. These are all due to the emphasis Jewish tradition places on family as a building block of society. Some Jewish parents will have strict views about their teenager not having a boyfriend/girlfriend from another religious faith. There may be a discomfort, reluctance or anger around comments on world politics and history, such as the Israel/Palestine conflict, the Holocaust and anti-Semitism. Tattoos are not approved by traditional Jewish law. However, like other issues within Judaism, this is changing and becoming more acceptable in some traditions.

By the bedside

It is common for Jewish patients to wear a *kippah* or *yarmulke* (skullcap), especially for prayer, but some people may wish to keep them on at all times. Patients or family members may also wear prayer shawls and use *tefillin* (phylacteries) (two small boxes containing scriptural verses and having leather straps, worn on the forehead and forearm) during morning prayer. Often patients will pull the curtains for privacy and use their bed for prayer. Quite often they won't use prayer rooms, but family may appreciate knowing where it is if they need a quiet space. There may be a request that at least ten people (a *minyan*) be allowed in the patient's room for prayer, and this should be facilitated where possible. It is highly unlikely that an interpreter will be required; however, some families may speak Yiddish or Hebrew.

Age-specific considerations
Babies

A boy is circumcized on his eighth day, when he is seven days old. For example, a boy born on Sunday, Sunday is his first day; Monday, when he is one day old, is his second day. So, Sunday, when he is on his eighth day and seven days old is the day of his circumcision. (Similarly, we are in the 21st century, but the years begin with 20, not 21.)

Infants

When weaning infants onto solid food, consider Jewish dietary laws and the restrictions, according to the family's wishes.

Children and teenagers

As a key part of maintaining Jewish identity, parents and family members may have to think about how their child can be involved in Jewish life and celebrate special events or rites of passage whilst in hospital. It might be important to maintain the Sabbath in hospital, despite the challenges to the environment the family may face (as they cannot lift objects or cook whilst participating in the Sabbath, the family may have to think creatively about how to celebrate the day of rest at the bedside). Jewish youth clubs and groups are important to many Jewish children and there may be ways to encourage the child to participate in Jewish learning and activities whilst in hospital. Some Jewish families may wish to teach their child Hebrew whilst in hospital as part of their ongoing Jewish education.

Working with the family

It is very important to ask the family how important their religion is to them. As with all faiths, some family members may have stronger beliefs than others, or may associate with the faith for cultural reasons only (i.e. they don't believe the teachings of the faith).

Sabbath, or the day of rest, is observed by many Jewish families from sundown on Friday evening to nightfall on Saturday evening, a time of 25 hours. Work forbidden on the Sabbath is 'creative work' rather than 'work' as understood in English. Thus, cooking is forbidden, and many Jewish families prepare food on Friday so that they do not cook on Saturday. Even switching on a light or signing one's name is considered creative work and is therefore avoided. In hospital it is

> **A CHAPLAIN'S VIEW**
> I think the most important thing to understand about Jewish chaplaincy is that we are here to support people in their faith, and therefore are not here to proselytize. Also that we pray in a universalist and encouraging way, for example 'We pray this in Your Holy Name.'

more difficult for a family to observe the Sabbath, particularly for the patient who may be asked to do things like lift their IV drip, which would break the Sabbath rules for some families. Additionally, the use of electrical items is discouraged for the Sabbath. So, it would be important for staff to ask a Jewish family before the Sabbath (starting Friday evening) if there is anything they can do to make the Sabbath easier, and for staff to try to understand why the Sabbath is important. Staff may not be able to contact family members on the Sabbath as many practising Jews do not answer the phone. However, the preservation of life takes precedence over the observance of the Sabbath.

Conducive environment

Ensuring that kosher food is available if requested is important. It is helpful to ask whether a rabbi is required when a child is approaching death. It is particularly important for many families that they are able to comply with Jewish traditions around purification of the body at death.

Views of suffering

There is a firm belief that G-d knows best and suffering is given for a reason – any attempt to second guess that reason is not appropriate as humans are not G-d. In terms of children, there is no fundamental difference. However, there is a belief that everyone is put on earth for a particular purpose, that there is something to fulfil.

A way to understand a child suffering and dying is to understand that they have completed their purpose and will have eternal life after death.

Suffering can also be seen as an atonement (reparation) for a sin, but the concept of punishment for particular actions is not part of the belief, as we cannot know God's reasons.

Attitudes to medical care

All Jews would understand that they have a responsibility to look after their bodies, minds and souls. This is because life is considered G-d given and therefore very precious – life should always be preserved no matter what, and this includes seeking appropriate medical treatment. There is a belief that doctors, nurses and other healthcare professionals are doing 'G-d's work'.

WHY ARE SOME CHILDREN BORN WITH LIFE-LIMITED CONDITIONS? A RABBI RESPONDS

Every birth is a gamble. A soul enters the world innocent and pure. But it may not stay that way. This world is a maze of diverging pathways, both good and evil, and the choice is ours which way we go... But in order to be protected from the potential evils of an earthly existence, they are sent down into a body that will not compromise their holiness. They enter this world in a form that is above sin, above evil. From a purely physical perspective we call them disabled or handicapped; from the perspective of the soul they are protected. They will never sin. Their sojourn in this world is often brief, and in terms of this world may seem sad. But they have retained their purity. (Rabbi Aron Moss, Nefesh Community, Sydney, Australia)[5]

Understanding illness and disease

Jews understand that the body, mind and spirit are all connected. For Jews, wellbeing is 'wholeness' or *shleimut*. Physical illness is understood to have psychological and spiritual effects. During prayers for the sick, Jews traditionally wish a sick person a *refuah shlema*, complete healing. Jews understand that illness is a part of life, and part of G-d's order, even if it cannot be understood. It is one of life's great mysteries.

Understanding mental illness

Recent research[6] has demonstrated that Jews, like many other people, understand mental illness to be caused by a range of factors. Some Jews attribute moral or social causes to mental illness (e.g. a bad character) without recognizing the genetic or biological causes. Beliefs about G-d's benevolence is an important factor for helping more traditional or Orthodox Jews cope with mental health problems.[7]

Pain management

Jews would welcome medical help with pain management but would also advocate religious interventions. Jews may recite Psalms that call out to G-d requesting comfort or help, for example Psalm 130, which begins 'Out of the depths I cry to you Lord.' Prayer may be very important.

Traditional healing and medicine

Modern Judaism incorporates prayer into scientific methods of cure and treatment. In ancient times, supernatural or mystical treatments, such as exorcism or spells, were suggested in the Talmudic literature. However, most Jews today reject this with the advance of scientific understanding of the body. Due to the interconnectedness of mind, body and spirit, many Jews would stress the importance of a good diet, healthy lifestyle and active spiritual life as part of staying well.

Understanding death

Jewish religious writings and philosophy focus on the importance of earthly life – doing G-d's duties and serving humanity. Therefore, there is little speculation about what will happen after death. There is no one view of the afterlife. However, there are beliefs about a time of judgement, and concepts of both heaven and hell. Views held on what happens after death may impact how a family want the body to be treated after death.

Preparing for death

If there is a chance the child could live, everything medically possible should be done, including putting them on life support. Once the child is on life support, taking the child off the life support might, depending upon the exact circumstances, be considered similar to killing under Jewish law. Therefore, no decision to remove life support should be taken before the family, if they so wish, have consulted their rabbi. There is no prohibition on transfusions.

When a child is approaching death:

- The family should be kept closely informed as religious practices need to be completed.

- The presence of a rabbi may be essential for many families.
- Special prayers and psalms may be said just before death, which should not be interrupted.
- One is not allowed to touch the body in the final breaths, as this could be considered to be hastening death.

Immediately after death:

- The body should not be touched after death except for removal of medical devices.
- There are some Jews who do not wish to look at the dead body.
- The Jewish burial society will help with the practical removal and preparation of the body.
- Photographs taken after death, which are sometimes called memorial photos, are unlikely to be wanted but – *ask, don't assume.*
- The body is considered to be sacred. The family and rabbi should be consulted beforehand if it should be necessary to move the body, so that advice can be sought before action is taken.
- Jews bury their dead as soon as possible after death, preferably on the same day. The family will therefore appreciate release of the body as soon as possible.
- Half an hour should be left before anything happens to the body.
- If the death has occurred as a result of a bleeding wound or injury, the bedclothes should be kept as many Jewish families consider it essential to bury blood alongside the body, as blood is seen as an important part of the body.

For many Jews is it vital that the body is never left alone. There may be a request to accompany the body until it is buried.

Organ donation and post-mortem

Organ and tissue donation are encouraged by some Jews as 'saving a life' is considered very important. However, respecting the dead may guide some to avoid donating certain organs. Additionally, according to some opinions, organs cannot be removed whilst there is still a heartbeat, as in Jewish law the person is still considered to be alive, despite an absence of other vital signs. This has implications for donating organs such as heart and lungs. Finally, families would be resistant to donate organs that are to be used for research, as this may not meet the criteria of 'saving a life' in the same way as an organ going to a recipient would. Families may consult their rabbi before making a decision.

Invasive post-mortems that pierce the skin are prohibited out of respect for the person who has died. The body needs to be buried in the same state it was born and Jews believe that the person has a right to rest in peace without their body being interfered with. It is permitted if there is absolutely no alternative, but family will be respectfully resistant. Some coroners allow MRI scans as an alternative to an invasive post-mortem.

Hospice care

There is no religious objection to hospice care. In fact hospice care may be encouraged, particularly where there is provision for Jewish hospices or specific religious needs.

Caring for the family after the death of their child

If staff wish to attend the funeral this will be well received but not expected. It will be at the cemetery, not the synagogue. Visiting the family is permitted, preferably within the first seven days. This is an intense period of mourning (*shiva*) that begins after the burial, and the family will have lots of visitors. Children can be incorporated into the grieving period as appropriate, and this will be led by the family.

Historically, the mourning of a neo-natal (before 30 days of life) death was not customary in Jewish law and ritual. Nowadays, for many Jewish families who have lost a baby, infant or child, a full *shiva* is expected. When mourning the death of their child, the father is relieved of the burden of 'being strong' for his wife and is permitted to mourn.

Garments are torn as an expression of grief, although this probably won't happen at the hospital. There are different stages of mourning for different family members, including a 7-day period, 30-day period,

11-month period, and a 1-year period for parents, with different prayers being said at each stage.

The funeral

In many Jewish communities, the *Chevra Kadisha*, a 'holy society', supervises funerals, helps to comfort the bereaved and makes sure that all Jewish laws and customs are followed for funeral ceremonies and rituals. Though they take place quickly, usually within 24 hours of death, Jewish funerals require preparation, a service and a mourning period, all in accordance with Jewish law and custom. A Jewish funeral director is usually contacted.

At the funeral a simple coffin will be used and you are unlikely to see flowers or hear singing. Jewish funerals take place at the graveside, sometimes with a service at the synagogue. In Orthodox Jewish funerals, it is likely that the body will be covered so that it cannot be viewed. Orthodox Jews are always buried, never cremated. For Reform Jews it is a matter of personal choice informed by religious belief. It is considered sacred to be buried in the ground. It is important that the gravestone that may be erected is simple. There is a Jewish law that states that Jews can only be buried in a Jewish cemetery.

For a stillborn baby, an infant or a child, the funeral is the same. The body should be buried within 24 hours (unless, in the case of a stillborn, the mother is not physically well enough to attend the funeral in which case an exception can be made). If the baby has not been named, it will usually be given a name at the graveside. There is a custom within Judaism (although not written in law) that pregnant women do not visit cemeteries as there is a belief that the distress experienced by the mother during such as visit will have a direct impact on the growing child.

Continuing bonds

There is no concept of continuing bonds – for example, the presence of the child still being felt or parents talking to child as if the child is still there. Religiously, the soul has moved on. This is very different to remembering the child, which is normal and important.

Key festivals

Specific rituals are associated with festivals, including fasting – the family or the rabbi will organize these, but it is good for staff to be aware that this might happen.

Passover: Celebrates the liberation of the Israelites who were led out of Egypt by Moses.

Rosh Hashanah (Jewish New Year): A two-day festival during which work is not permitted.

Yom Kippur (Day of Atonement): The holiest of days in the Jewish calendar.

Sukkot (Festival of Booths, Feast of Tabernacles): A Biblical Jewish harvest festival holiday which lasts seven to eight days.

Hanukkah: Festival of lights celebrating the miracle of the Temple oil never running out.

PASSOVER – A CHAPLAIN'S EXPERIENCE

A Jewish rabbi told me that it is probably best not to try to offer any hospital commemoration of Passover. It is such a family- and home-centered event that we could not possibly host anything that would make a Jewish family feel anything but loss by being hospitalized at that time. I wonder if hospitals in areas with larger Jewish populations have a different experience. Was this only one rabbi's opinion? One year during Christian Holy Week when we held a Christian service, a Jewish employee asked me why we didn't hold anything for Passover. When I told him of the rabbi's advice, this employee thought it over and agreed with him. (Rev Mark Bartel, Orlando, Florida)

Celebrating Rosh Hashanah and Yom Kippur

Rosh Hashanah is the Jewish New Year and is a commemoration of both creation and the Day of Judgement. It is a time to reflect on priorities in life and look back at the past year, asking forgiveness for things done wrong. Yom Kippur is the most sacred day in the Jewish calendar and means the Day of Atonement, and often Jews will fast on that day for 25 hours. The ten days between the two festivals are known as the Days of Awe, Yamim Nora'im, and this is a period of putting things right with G-d and other people. Traditionally, apples dipped in honey are eaten to celebrate Rosh Hashanah and apple-shaped cards can be made to wish people a happy Jewish New Year. For older children and young people this period can be used to reflect, for example:

- What's the most meaningful thing in my life?
- Who in my life means the most to me? How often do I let them know this?
- What are the significant things I've achieved in the past year?
- What do I hope to achieve next year and in my life generally?

Cut-out paper figures can be used on which to write the answers to these questions.

Further reading

Musleah, R. and Klayman, M. (2000) *Sharing Blessings: Children's Stories for Exploring the Spirit of the Jewish Holidays.* Woodstock, VT: Jewish Lights Publishing.

Notes

1   Extract printed with kind permission from an interview with Rabbi Lord Jonathan Sacks in *The Texas Jewish Post,* 24 April 2014. Available at www.rabbisacks.org/news/interview-texas-jewish-post, accessed on 24 November 2014.

2   See the Kaplan Center website for further information about these themes, www.kaplancenter.org

3   Kalish, N. (2013) 'Jewish Healthcare Chaplaincy: Professionalizing Spiritual Caregiving.' In J. Levin and M.F. Prince (eds) *Judaism and Health: A Handbook of Practical, Professional and Scholarly Resources,* Woodstock, VT: Jewish Lights Publishing, p.78.

4   Babylonian *Talmud, Shabbat* 152, 119.

5   Moss, A. 'Why does G-d create severely handicapped babies?' Available at www.chabad.org/library/article_cdo/aid/362221/jewish/Why-Does-G-d-Create-Severely-Handicapped-Babies.htm, accessed on 16 January 2015. Aron Moss is rabbi of the Nefesh Community in Sydney, Australia, and is a frequent contributor to Chabad.org. Reprinted with permission from Chabad.org.

6   Pirutinsky, S., Rosen, D.D., Shapiro Safran, R. and Rosmarin, D.H. (2010) 'Do medical models of mental illness relate to increased or decreased

stigmatization of mental illness among Orthodox Jews?' *The Journal of Nervous and Mental Disease 198*, 7, 508–512.

7   Rosmarin, D.H., Pirutinsky, S., Pargament, K.I. and Krumrei, E.J. (2009) 'Are religious beliefs relevant to mental health among Jews?' *American Psychological Association 1*, 3, 180–190.

6

CARE OF A MUSLIM CHILD AND FAMILY

Zamir Hussain and Madeleine Parkes

Introduction to Islam

Muslims follow the religion of Islam. Islam literally means peace through submission to the one God called Allah. Islam is an Abrahamic monotheistic religion, meaning it shares a history with Christianity and Judaism and believes in one God. Islam is a holistic way of life. Its laws govern every aspect of life: social, political, personal, spiritual and psychological. Islam has no formal clergy or hierarchy. However, Muslims are supported by scholars learned in Islamic sciences and the Arabic language.

21ST-CENTURY ISLAM

Islam is the second largest religion in the world after Christianity. There are approximately 1.66 billion Muslims in the world and it is the fastest growing religion. Islamic jurisprudence, or the philosophy of law, derives practical laws by using *ijtihad*, which means using logic to create rules from original sources in order to address contemporary situations and problems. It draws upon *qiyas*: anology; *ihtishan*: legal presumptions; *urf*: custom; and *ijma*: consensus and is thus adaptable for any time and place, and is applicable, for example, to the issue of organ donation.

Muslims believe in a line of Prophets starting from Adam and including Moses and Jesus as conveyors of God's Message but not as divine themselves. The following information is given as a guide to culture, religion and spirituality. It is important to use this as a starting point, and when working with a Muslim child and family always remember to *ask* about their beliefs and practices. Do not assume you know everything as every Muslim is unique.

Beliefs and rituals

The Islamic name for God is Allah. This name has no plural. Muslims believe God is the Creator and Sustainer, God is all knowing. God never tires or sleeps, God needs no subsistence, God cannot be imagined by the human mind. Thus Muslims are not encouraged to make mental or physical representations of God. He is known through the 99 Beautiful Names (*Asma al-Husna*), which describe His Attributes – these all appear in the *Quran*, the Islamic holy book. Muslims will use these attributes to explore the essence of God. Examples include the Loving, the Merciful, the Creator, the Life-Giver, the Provider. Muslims believe that God is always near. Allah is also an all-powerful God who hears one's prayers and thoughts and is considered to be 70 times more loving than a mother. Muslims believe that people are God's representatives on earth and that this life is a preparation for the eternal life in the hereafter. Muslims are required to follow the five obligatory pillars and the six basic beliefs.

Five Pillars:

1. *Shahada*: declaration of faith
2. *Salah*: five daily ritual prayers
3. *Saum*: fasting in the month of Ramadan
4. *Zakat*: welfare/charity
5. *Hajj*: pilgrimage to Makkah.

Six basic beliefs:

1. *Tawhid*: oneness of Allah
2. *Angels and the unseen world*
3. *Belief in the Messengers and Prophets*
4. *The Revealed books*
5. *Day of Judgement*
6. *Qadr*: predestination.

These obligations are only for adult, sane and able Muslims. Children are considered adults in terms of religious duties from puberty or from the age of nine for females and 15 for males.

Concept of worship in Islam

Every act of life can be a form of worship if one is doing it for the purpose of pleasing God and fulfilling one's responsibilities to self and creation – for example, eating can be an act of worship if done whilst showing gratitude for the provision of food and the purpose of gaining energy for good works and health. Thus, looking after a sick child would be an act of worship as one is looking after a needy creation of God. In fact a believer's whole life can be an act of worship, all depending on the intention and sincerity.

Muslims believe in the Prophet Muhammad as God's last messenger to whom the holy book, the *Quran*, was revealed through the angel Gabriel. Muslims see the Prophet Muhammad as a role model, an embodiment of the message of the *Quran*, and an intercessor on the Day of Judgement. They often try to emulate his behaviour and lifestyle. This would be called following the *sunnah* (tradition), for example the beard is a *sunnah* of the Prophet. Further to this they have a great love and reverence for him and consider sending peace and salutations upon him as a source of great religious and spiritual importance.

The *Quran* is considered to be the last and final testament, a source of guidance and healing for mankind. The *Quran* is accepted as the literal speech of God in book form, revealed in an earthly language of Arabic, although translations exist in many languages. Muslims all over the world will learn the *Quran* in Arabic even though they may not be taught to understand the language. Many Muslims also memorize the *Quran* and will be known as *hafiz* (one in whose heart the *Quran* is protected). Muslims will treat the *Quran* with great respect in that they will only wish to touch it in the state of ritual purity.

Denominations

The majority of the world's Muslims are *Sunni* Muslims, with a minority following *Shia* Islam. Many beliefs are the same across the two groups, the major difference being debates around who succeeded the Prophet

Muhammad. There are very few practical differences that you will observe in a hospital setting. You may see *Shia* Muslims praying with a clay block, which is considered a sacred reminder of a holy place. *Shia* Muslims also have an organized hierarchy of religious leaders, which may impact the decision to bring in a representative from the faith to advise on religious and spiritual issues. *Shia* Muslims also have an additional two pillars of faith concerning purity (of mind, body and action) and the concept of struggle (*jihad*) towards Allah despite all challenges, a concept that *Sunni* Muslims would also recognize but do not consider a core pillar. Orthodox Islam recognizes Sufism as a mystical and mysterious denomination of Islam and is respected.

Names and greetings

Muslims are encouraged to greet all other Muslims by saying *Assalamu alaikum* (peace be with you) both on meeting and leaving. The reply would be *Wa alaikum salaam* (peace be upon you also). Muslims from the Indian subcontinent may say *Kuda hafis* or *Allah hafiz* (may Allah keep you in His protection) for goodbye.

Muslim names are usually Arabic in origin and easily recognizable by the Muslim or trained eye. A child should be named promptly at birth or by the seventh day. Sometimes names are changed if they are deemed to be having a negative influence on someone's life. Muslims are often named after the Prophets or pious people or after noteworthy and beautiful characteristics. Some names are used as titles such as Muhammad in honour of the Prophet. In such cases the second name will become the personal name. Many Muslim cultures do not have the tradition of a family surname, but may include the father's first name. Women are not required to change their name after marriage.

Family life

Marriage and family life are important in Islam. Muslims often live within an extended family structure and place high value on family life. There is often a hierarchy of the elders, who are treated with great respect. All relatives do not necessarily live together but links between them are reinforced by Islamic law. Parents have great honour and respect; the *Quran* encourages kindness to parents. Parents are to be obeyed and respected. Taking care of parents is a duty and a key to

Paradise. Causing them distress and pain is a block to Paradise, which only they can remove through forgiveness.

The concept of *ummah* (nation) includes all Muslims as one family. Culture plays a major role and will vary amongst Muslims. Some cultural practices may override or be confused with religious teachings by some families. However, the golden rule always applies, no matter how much factual knowledge you have read – *ask, don't assume.*

Regarding family planning, childless couples and infertility can be a problematic situation in most Muslim cultures. Artificial insemination and in-vitro fertilization (IVF) are acceptable but surrogacy and sperm donations are prohibited. The soul of the child is believed by most Muslims to enter the foetus at 120 days, and some sources put this earlier, whereupon the foetus has full human rights. Thus abortion is not allowed unless the mother's life is in danger or there are specific extreme circumstances such as rape. Some jurists may allow abortion in the case of serious foetal abnormalities, or imminent baby death upon birth, or risk to the mother's mental health.

Muslims will often be affiliated to a particular *masjid*, or mosque, according to their origins and religious viewpoints. They may or may not attend regular congregations. However, they will often prefer to take the opinion and advice of a particular *imam* (leader) or scholar or school of thought. Some masjids also have a *madrassa* (Islamic school). Muslim children will often start attending *madrassa* after school or on weekends by the age of four to learn the *Quran* in Arabic and religious studies. For many children this will continue into their teenage years.

WOMEN IN FAMILY LIFE

Men and women have equal status in Islam. The *Quran* acknowledges the physical differences and other sources state that the best men are those who are good to their wives, and Paradise lies at the feet of the mother. A woman has rights to inherit and to own property; to choose her husband; to gain custody of her children; to divorce; to sexual and emotional fulfilment; to an education; and to work.

There have been exceptional female Muslim figures throughout Islamic history. Cultural practices and male dominant societies take away some of these rights.

And for women are rights over men similar to those of men over women. (*Quran* 2: 226)

Languages

There will be many languages spoken by Muslims as they will come from all over the world. Muslims from the Indian subcontinent will speak mainly Urdu, Hindi and Arabic. Farsi and some African languages may also be popular, and English may be spoken as a second language by some. There will be different dialects and variations within these main groups. For the younger generation growing up in English-speaking countries they may have difficulty in communicating with non-English speaking elders and grandparents.

The Quranic Arabic language holds a special status in Islam and is read from right to left, although numbers are left to right. It was the language of the Prophet. The *Quran* is considered more meritorious to be recited in Arabic, and the daily prayers are always said in Arabic. Thus, all learned Muslims will know some Arabic to read and pray but may not always understand what it means.

Stories and attitudes to children

Islam gives great credence to children's rights. In fact these start even before conception, in that a spouse should be chosen who would make a good parent. Children have a right to a good name; a two-year nursing period; a right to sustenance and a good environment; equal gifts and treatment with siblings; a good education and good manners; the mother's custody or the next of kin if the mother is not capable; and safety and security. There is a prohibition against child labour, abuse and exploitation, and children have inheritance rights. A pregnant or nursing mother has rights. A child born out of wedlock is not blameworthy but innocent and pure.

CHILDREN IN ISLAM

A child becomes an adult at puberty or by the age of 15 when religious obligations become compulsory. Generally, rules of modesty and gender apply after the age of ten. Children are considered a blessing and a trust from God. Males and females have equal status.

Children are also a source of blessing in terms of the hereafter in that the parent will benefit from the child's good works and prayers and a young child that dies before the parent will become a means of the parents entering Paradise without any judgement.

Taking care of a child with a disability or serious illness is seen as a source of great blessing and reward for the carer. For this reason, some Muslims may not wish to receive extra help from outside agencies, perhaps feeling that they are giving up their reward, or are not doing their duty, and may suffer physically and emotionally through stress and exhaustion. The Prophet Muhammad had great love and compassion for all children and taught others to be kind, loving and benevolent to children. He would often give children a ride on his mount when returning home.

A story about the Prophet's son

All of the Prophet's sons died in infancy. When Ibrahim took his last breaths, the Prophet could not control his grief as tears were flowing from his eyes. The Prophet's friend Abdur-Rahman bin Awf said, 'O the Messenger of God, even you weep!' The Prophet said, 'O bin Awf, this is mercy.' Then he wept more and said, 'The eyes shed tears and the heart grieves, and we will not say except what pleases our Lord, O Ibrahim! Indeed I am grieved by your separation. If I did not know that I will see you again indeed my heart would break.' This story may bring some solace to parents whose child is ill or dying, as they know that the Prophet Muhammed would have experienced sadness and grief in the same way.

Role models

Muslims take the Prophet Muhammad as the ultimate role model and teach their children through his example of conduct, manner, dress and practice what it means to achieve the ideal of human perfection. They also have the great companions and figures from history, both male and female. Each Muslim is encouraged to be a good role model and example to others.

Care of Muslim patients and their families in hospital

Every Muslim will differ slightly in the details of their beliefs and practices, so the information given here should be seen as a guide from which to ask further questions.

Key points:

- A peaceful environment free from images of humans or animals will be welcomed by a Muslim family.

- Daily prayers form an important part of the religious life of a Muslim family and should be facilitated.

- There are significant dietary laws in Islam and several prohibited products that could affect the choice of medication. In addition, there are important modesty rules concerning dress and cleanliness.

- Children are encouraged to follow Islam from a young age, but have personal responsibility for their faith after puberty.

- Follow personal family wishes at all times, although be aware of the decision-making hierarchy within the family and the use of a religious leader to help make decisions about healthcare.

- Children should be conversed with in a respectful way. They may be reluctant to talk about their personal beliefs and practices.

Food and prohibited products

Food can be categorized as *halal* (permissible) or *haram* (not permissible). All vegetables, nuts, pulses and fish with scales are *halal* (there is a difference of opinion regarding other sea creatures). Meat slaughtered in a *halal* way is permissible. Forbidden is the pig and any porcine products. Blood products and alcohol are also strongly prohibited. There may be a fear of hospital food not being *halal*. There may also be a wish to provide certain foods and herbs which are seen to have both healing and preventative qualities, and culturally sensitive food for those accustomed to a different cuisine. Some Muslims will not wish to use alcohol gel, as alcohol is considered impure. Prohibited substances may be used for necessary medication and to save life if no alternative is available.

During the month of Ramadan, Muslims abstain from food, drink and sexual intercourse from dawn to dusk. Fasting also involves avoidance of negative behaviour and habits, and cultivation of good. Oral medication nullifies the fast, whilst non-nutritious injections (intravenous, intramuscular and subcutaneous), eye and ear drops, and blood taken through thumb prick or intravenous means do not break the fast. Children under the age of puberty, those who are not of sound mind or who have a long-term incurable illness are totally exempt. There are also concessions for the sick, pregnant, breast-feeding mothers and travellers. Some Muslims may insist on fasting, even though they are exempt, to the detriment of their health under the impression that they will be rewarded for such actions. However, Islam teaches to take concessions and not harm one's health.

Modesty and hygiene

Care provided by staff of the same gender is preferable for teenagers and young adults in order to preserve modesty. Generally, children under the age of ten do not require this, although ideas about modesty may be strong and even young children may not want to change in front of others.

Both men and women are required to cover their *awra* (nakedness). This is for both modesty and protection. For a male this will mean the navel to the knee and for the female most of her body except the face, hands and feet. Some may consider these parts also as part of her *awra* depending on interpretation and sometimes cultural practices. Sometimes eye contact may be avoided by some Muslims when talking to a member of the opposite sex. A young woman may be encouraged to wear a *hijab* (hair covering) in front of non-related males. She may dress as she pleases in the privacy of her own home. The *nikab* (face veil) may be removed in front of female staff. Not all Muslim women choose to wear the *hijab*, and fewer still wear the *nikab*.

Ritual washing is a key practice in Islam. Running water is to be used where possible. Blood, urine and faeces on the body, clothing or surroundings will render them impure. Nails should be cut and pubic and under-arm hair is to be removed. A *ghusl* (ritual bath) will be required after menstruation, post-natal bleeding or emission of any sexual fluid. Muslims may wish to bathe on Fridays as this is the Islamic holy day. Ablution is required for certain acts of worship and to remain in a spiritually pure and protected state. Ablution facilities should be provided near the Muslim prayer room. Those not able to wash can do a symbolic purification called *tayumum* consisting of wiping hands over a natural surface such as a stone and then wiping over the face, hands and arms. Children will participate in this ritual washing prior to prayer. Good dental hygiene is also very important. Traditionally, Muslims will use a *miswak* which was also the *sunnah* (practice) of the Prophet. The *miswak* is a natural stick from the Peelu tree and can be used without toothpaste.

Taboos

Amongst Muslims of many cultures, domestic and sexual abuse is a taboo topic. Very little data exist on the incidence of abuse in Muslim families, and those who have spoken out have often delayed reporting the abuse experienced due to social pressure and stigma. Sexuality is a complex subject in Islam. The *Quran* and other sources are very clear about the joy and importance of sex within marriage and the rights of both men and women to have sexual fulfilment. Sex outside of marriage is generally not acceptable, which can create issues within a family if a teenager in hospital is sexually active. Sex education for teenagers can cause some discomfort amongst practising Muslim parents who may have stricter views of sex and sexual morality. The *Quran* celebrates human diversity but does not explicitly refer to same-sex couples. Traditional Islamic law forbids homosexuality and considers it sinful. In some Islamic countries homosexuality is punishable by death, or is illegal. Some countries with high populations of Muslims tolerate or have legalized same-sex relationships.

Some young Muslims may experience bullying and stigma around their culture and religion. Unhelpful media portrayals of extremist Islam may add to this. Some young Muslims may be struggling to incorporate Muslim ideals and teachings into the Western culture in which they live. Some of their decisions and actions about the way they dress, their interactions with friends of the opposite sex and peer pressures around drugs and alcohol may come as a surprise to their parents and family members, especially if there are high expectations for the young person to live an Islamic way of life. In a 2011 European research study it was found that eating disorders and body dissatisfaction were twice as high amongst Muslim teenagers as amongst their Christian peers.[1] Islam teaches that food is a blessing and that one should not do harm to one's body.

By the bedside

Items that a child in hospital may have by their bed include whatever the individual and the family would find most beneficial in helping to create a positive and peaceful environment.

The *Quran*, the holy book of Islam, may be beside the bed. The *Quran* is often covered with a cloth and placed on a high place. Muslims believe that angels surround one who is reading the *Quran*. The *Quran* will be read on a daily basis if possible. Most Muslims will endeavour to complete a reading during Ramadan. It will be used in prayer gatherings, and certain verses will be used to promote healing; as a way out of difficulties; for particular aims; for protection and worship. Muslims will also treat the Bible with respect, in the belief that it also contains some revelation. Certain verses of the *Quran* may be displayed around the sick bed or worn in amulets.

Prayer beads and counting devices may be used to help engage in numbered or free repetitions of the Names or Attributes of God; salutations upon the Prophet or Quranic scripture to help healing and invoke peace in the reader. They can also be used to help focus on remembering God. Some Muslims may not agree with the use of these means.

You may find many visitors around the bed. Visiting the sick is a duty of every Muslim and one will be questioned about this on the Day of Judgement. There are great blessings in visiting the sick, and prayers of the sick are answered. To be prevented from visiting may cause distress to the visitor in view of not being able to fulfil the obligation, receive blessings and offer support and empathy. Islam, however, rewards according to intention, so if prevention is necessary then the visitor will receive the good outcomes even though he or she was prevented from visiting.

A sick child may wish to practise their faith in hospital. They may require gender segregation after the age of ten and adhere to the Islamic dress code. They may want to continue some *madrassa* (Islamic school) work, have *halal* food and they may wish to perform the ritual prayers and know the *Qibla* (direction for prayer). Listening to or reading the *Quran* may also be a comforting and important practice.

Every effort should be made to use a professional translator if one is needed, not a family member of the patient. Where practical, a chaplain may be able to offer translation skills. If using a family member to translate, be very mindful that they are hearing the news you are telling them for the first time and may not fully understand what is being said. If they do understand they may not be able to find the most accurate words to translate the information into – this is particularly true for unfamiliar medical terminology or concepts – and they should be invited to clarify their understanding with you. A religious leader may be called in to help with ethical and moral decisions which have a religious impact.

RESPECTING THE *QURAN*

- Try not to touch the *Quran* if possible, or place any objects on top of it, or place it on the floor.
- Do not remove the *Quran* without permission.
- Some Muslims may not wish to turn their backs towards it.
- Be careful whilst handling any amulets that are worn as they may contain verses of the *Quran*.
- Be aware that many Muslims may wish to have an audio of the *Quran* playing and will find this very comforting.
- Cover the *Quran* in cloth when handling the Arabic version if this is possible. The Arabic version should be placed on a high shelf.

Age-specific considerations

Babies

Shortly after birth the child is given *thaneek*, something sweet upon the tongue such as honey or mashed date. This was a custom of the Prophet and the sweetness can alleviate some of the trauma of birth. The *adhan* and *iqama* (call to prayer) is said in to the child's ears, so that the first words they hear are calling to the worship of the one God. The hair is also shaved soon after birth. Traditionally, a sacrifice of animals ceremony known as *aqeeqa* is performed and the meat is distributed. Breast-feeding is of religious merit and highly recommended. Male circumcision is among the rites of Islam and is a tradition of the Prophet Abraham. It will provide health benefits in the child's life. Female circumcision is practised in some predominantly African cultures; however, it is not accepted as part of Islam and is considered a violation of the child's human rights.

Children

During a particularly long illness or stay in hospital, falling behind in studies set by the Islamic school (*madrassa*) could be a cause of distress for the family. Some provision through the Muslim chaplain or religious education teaching from school teachers could help. Depending on the influence of their family, Muslim children may be dressed in Western clothes or more traditional dress. Covering the body for modesty purposes, including wearing head coverings, usually occurs after puberty.

Teenagers

Issues surrounding gender segregation (an ideal for most Muslims) becomes a factor for teenagers on a hospital ward. Ideally, adolescent men and women should not be on a mixed ward in order to preserve modesty and dignity. Muslim parents may encourage their teenager to socialize with fellow Muslims in hospital where possible, and to be respectful to their peers.

Working with the family

Muslims are often brought up with the knowledge that families will look after each other at times of distress and illness, and believe that there is great reward as well as duty to do this. You may find extended family as well as immediate family around the bed. Decisions will often be made in consultation with the main decision-maker, often the head of the family and not necessarily the next of kin. It may be useful to identify the key people to save time and repetition. An Islamic verdict may be required for decision-making – time should be allowed for this and the Muslim chaplain can offer support and advice in this situation. Culture plays a major role and will vary

RELIGIOUS INVOLVEMENT IN DECISION-MAKING

The need to fulfil religious requirements may be heightened during times of stress. Muslims may wish to get a religious verdict before making any major decisions and will often turn to faith for answers and guidance. They may want to become more vigilant in performing religious duties such as *salah* (ritual) prayer, fasting, etc. A Muslim chaplain or *imam* may be able to offer support and guidance.

amongst Muslims. Some cultural practices may override or be confused with religious teachings by some families.

Conducive environment

The colour green is spiritually significant. Quranic scripture and other objects such as amulets will be appreciated. Some Muslims are often uncomfortable with pictures or images of human beings or animals, especially with the eyes showing. This may include dolls and toys. Drawings of these images could become an issue for Muslim children. However, the majority view is that drawing is allowed as long as the images do not depict nudity or other indecent representations, and are not three-dimensional sculptures or glorified. Images were initially prohibited to prevent idol worship and establish monotheism. Good smells are also believed to increase spiritual and positive energy, and have a profound effect on the soul, which yearns for beauty. Traditionally, oils and woods are burnt often in the form of incense sticks and the smoke perfumes the room and clothing. The limitations of using these in hospital may have to be explained.

Views of suffering

Affliction and tribulation are seen as part of God's plan for the soul during its probationary period on earth. Suffering is not seen as a punishment or a result of God's anger, but rather a sign of His love and mercy and a means of raising one's spiritual status, resolve and character, as well as a means of bringing one closer to God. God tests those He loves and tests are according to spiritual ranks. Thus the Prophets were the most severely tested. The suffering of a child is a test for the parents and will also raise the spiritual status of the child in the hereafter. However, some Muslims may see suffering as a punishment of sins. Muslims are taught to turn to God and to adopt *sabr* (endurance, perseverance, acceptance and withholding oneself from utter despair). *Sabr* involves believing in Divine decree and knowing that all is from God's wisdom and that good will come from it. The benefits of suffering do not mean that it must be endured without seeking relief. Every effort must be made to find a cure, both medical and spiritual, and this must be implemented. However, if a discomfort does not interfere with daily worship and duties, and does not risk one's life or health, then one may choose to accept it without seeking a cure.

Purposes of suffering

Suffering can be seen as having many different purposes for Muslims, including:

- a test of faith

- a means to Paradise and atonement of sins

- to reinstate one's relationship with God

- to give a chance to re-evaluate one's life and journey

- to become more empathetic towards others

- to become grateful for and appreciate what is good in one's life

- to know that God is close, and to turn to Him

- to realize the transient nature of this life

- to reduce the tendency to materialism, and focus on the hereafter

- as a remedy against spiritual weakness.

Attitudes to medical care

Western medicine has replaced the core of healthcare systems in Islamic countries. However, most Muslims will not dismiss either natural or synthetic medicine. The challenge will be to define the interrelationship of how they may work together or when one may be more useful than the other. 'There is no disease that Allah has created, except that He also has created its treatment' (Bukhari).[2]

Islamic teaching prompted Muslims to exert themselves in all fields of knowledge, including medical knowledge. They built upon existing knowledge and pioneered great advancements. This resulted in amazing leaps in standards of human healthcare, including the first hospitals, advancement in chemistry, pharmaceutical drugs, surgical equipment and techniques, and many procedures that are still in use today.

Prophetic medicine refers to the words and actions of the Prophet Muhammad with regard to disease, treatment and care of patients, and covers preventative, curative and mental wellbeing. It includes spiritual cures, surgical treatments, the use of products such as honey, yoghurt, black seed and other natural products, as well as cupping[3] and preventative measures such as quarantine, personal and dental hygiene, moderation in eating habits and dietary laws. Prophetic medicine in essence is holistic medicine. Muslims hold prophetic medicine in great esteem for its doctrinal and theological value, holding it as timeless and sacred. Prophetic medicine is, however, a distinct form of Islamic medicine which later developed under scientific and analytical observations, although prophetic medicine has also been tested by these methods.

Understanding illness and disease

Muslims understand disease and its cures to be the wisdom and work of Allah. The Islamic holistic way of life results in setting health and disease within a religious and spiritual framework. Disease can be both physical and spiritual. Islam advocates the importance of the health of one's inner being – the heart, mind and soul as well as the body. Islam ascertains rights to the body such as cleanliness, wholesome food, exercise, rest and avoidance of what may harm. The health of the heart, mind and soul will be promoted by living a God conscience (being aware that God is watching one's actions and inner thoughts and intentions) and righteous life (living under the moral and practical guidance from Islamic teachings). In some Muslim cultures there is a lack of understanding about physical illness in children. For example, for some parents of South Asian origin, they did not know that cancer could affect children or that there were treatment options for it.[4] Careful explanations of the diagnosis and prognosis are especially important in this case.

Understanding mental illness

The Islamic perspective does not treat mental illness as a stigma but as a genuine illness. Muslims were amongst the first to build mental health hospitals. However, culture and individual attitude often play a major role. There may be some prejudiced and discriminatory views against people with mental illness, and often people may not wish to accept the fact that their child may have mental health issues. Mental illness can be culturally attributed to *jinn* (spirit) possession, the evil eye or black magic. There may be a delay in seeking medical help as parents or carers decide to seek spiritual cures, and the disease may reach an advanced stage by the time medical treatment is sought. Medical diagnosis may not be accepted whilst still holding on to the belief that the symptoms have been caused by untoward forces and patients may refuse drug treatments. Spiritual cures do exist; however, people may become victims of unscrupulous 'healers' who exploit vulnerable people financially. Muslims may feel that they are not being understood or find it difficult to explain their beliefs about mental illness to non-Muslims.

Suicide is considered a major sin in most Islamic schools of thought, as it was taught by the Prophet Muhammad that one's life is a trust from God, so taking one's life is against God's will and the sanctity of life. However, it will not be considered a sin if the individual's mental state comes into question. For a young person who has committed suicide, fellow Muslims would be encouraged to pray for God's mercy on behalf of them. There will be questions about why the person's trust and belief in God had failed them. However, they are also encouraged not to judge the person.

A CHAPLAIN'S EXPERIENCE

A 14-year-old girl was admitted to the mental health unit. She was found to be wearing a black thread around her waist and wrist. When asked by the staff what it was, she replied that she did not know.

Staff contacted the Muslim chaplain, who explained that this could be a talisman worn to ward off the evil energies to which the family may be attributing her mental state. It transpired that the girl did know what it was but was not saying for fear of being ridiculed or misunderstood.

Pain management

A Muslim child would be encouraged to manage pain through prayer and knowing that others are praying for him or her. There are certain prayers and attributes of God which are repeated for healing and peace.

These can be read and blown on the child or said over water that is then given to drink. There are no restrictions for necessary medication even if it contains prohibited products such as pig and alcohol if no alternative is available at the time.

SPIRITUAL SUPPORT DURING SUFFERING

On no soul does Allah place a burden greater than it can bear. (*Quran* (94: 5–6)

Verily, after hardship comes ease. Verily, with hardship there is relief. (*Quran* 94: 6)

Traditional healing and medicine

Traditional Islamic medicine expounds the concept of innate harmony. Elements and temperaments are broken into four constitutions of dry, cold, hot and humid. Foods are also believed to have hot or cold temperaments, and atmospheric climate will also influence individual health. Each person has an innate temperament which will affect them in a different way and thus the treatment, the foods they eat and climate they live in will have an individual effect. Medical cures consist of natural and pharmaceutical products, as well as quarantine and cleanliness. Muslims have also employed spiritual cures such as the power of prayer. In addition to personal prayers, they will often ask others for prayer; in particular, they will contact friends and relatives as well as mosques for prayers. There may be gatherings for prayer and reading the holy scripture in the hope of invoking a miraculous healing. *Zam Zam* is holy water from the holy city of Makkah used for healing and blessing. Muslims will often want to administer this water to the sick and dying and partake from it for blessings.

Understanding death

Muslims believe that the time of death is predestined. Death is seen as a detachment of the soul from the body, and change of state and dimension of existence. Upon death the soul leaves the body and crosses over to the eternal life. Indeed, it is a joyful occasion for the righteous soul, 'Death is a gift to the believer' (Bukhari). Children are innocent and pure, and thus will have no judgement at the time of death. The souls of children, including those that are stillborn or miscarried, enter into the *barzakh* (intermediate world) into the care of the Prophet Abraham. Here they have a happy and prosperous life. Likened to a great kindergarten or nursery of heaven, parents of a dying child understand that their child is going to be taken care of by God and that they will meet again. These children will intercede for their parents on the Day of Judgement and take them into Paradise; the parents will therefore have no judgement.

Preparing for death

Families may not want the child to know of a grave diagnosis. This will be due to the fear that the patient may give up hope. Families and carers will also be reluctant to accept the seriousness of a diagnosis, as faith and hope in God's mercy and healing are fundamental parts of Islam. Terminal illness in particular causes a communal response and for the community to visit the sick and respond to the needs of the family. It is also a duty for Muslims to support the dying and their family. You may find a large number of visitors around the time of death, particularly as death is seen as a communal event and it is important to make peace with the dying. It is considered a good sign to die on a Thursday or Friday and during Ramadan. Muslims consider death in the holy cities of Makkah and Madina to be a desirable death.

Death is not a taboo subject and children are often made aware of the Islamic belief that this life is a preparation for the hereafter, and that death is inevitable. Thus, children are often not excluded in the rituals for the deceased. They will, for example, be encouraged to be at the funerals. A dying child will be told of the love and mercy of God; of the beautiful existence that awaits; that those who love one another will meet again in the eternal life after death; and that the separation will be short.

In hospital, the Muslim chaplain may explore death through activities that facilitate discussion about inner fears and concerns, and help the family to find ways of making the most of their time together.

When a child is approaching death:

- In Islam it is preferable for the child to die at home, surrounded by family and friends. For some Muslim families, dying in hospital, in a sterile environment, being cared for by strangers is not ideal.

- The dying child will be given the holy water of *Zam Zam*.

- The child is encouraged to repeat the *shahada* (declaration of faith) in whatever capacity they can.

- The chapter Yasin from the *Quran* is often recited around the bed. This is believed to help the soul leave more peacefully.

- The bed is turned so that the child's face or right side is turned towards Makkah.

- There is no wailing or loud crying.

- The last sounds that are heard are of the melodious recitation of the *Quran* and the affirmation of faith.

- Where possible, the room is perfumed.

Immediately after death:

- The eyes and mouth are closed. Sometimes a cloth or bandage is tied around the jaw and head to keep the mouth closed if needed.

- The arms and legs are straightened, and sometimes ankles are tied to keep the legs straight. This is for aesthetic reasons and for ease of washing, shrouding and burial.

- The face is kept facing slightly to the right, as the body will be buried facing Makkah.

- The body is completely covered by a cloth.

- It is not necessary for the body to be washed by hospital staff as this will not constitute ritual washing. It can be wiped down and made presentable.

- A local funeral director will be called once the body is ready for release. Arrangements will be made for the washing and shrouding of the body, funeral prayers and burial.

Organ donation and post-mortem

Organ donation is a controversial issue. The majority of Islamic jurists allow for organ donation; however, many Muslims will be reluctant to donate. They may believe that the body will feel pain because of their interpretation of a sacred text that states that any violation dealt to a body whether alive or not is equal. Also the body is seen as a trust from God. Post-mortems are allowed if required by law. However, for the same reasons as organ donation there may be strong reluctance. When a post-mortem is required, Muslims would much prefer an MRI as an alternative to a surgical post-mortem. Procedures that expose the body, such as organ donation and post-mortem, are also not desirable due to the requirement to keep the body covered.

Hospice care

Taking care of a sick child is seen as a source of great blessing and reward for the carer. Some Muslim families may be reluctant to consider receiving extra help from outside agencies. They may have misconceptions about what a hospice is. A visit and exploration of the facilities may serve to alleviate fears and show the benefits of hospice care.

Caring for the family after the death of their child

The death of a child will be followed by a three-day period set aside for the family to receive condolences. This may be in the mosque or at home. Food will be provided for the family, and prayers and Quranic readings will take place. Condolence prayers will be repeated to the bereaved as a form of solace. There are no formal dress codes; however, modest clothing is preferred. Condolences will consist of enjoinment of *sabr* (God's will; patience, forbearance and perseverance) and Islamic teachings as well as prayers and other support. Grief and mourning are individual and unique experiences; expressions of grief may be culturally influenced.

CONDOLENCES

Muslims will repeat part of a verse from the *Quran*: 'Truly to Allah we belong and to Him is our return' (*Quran* 156). This is said upon any disturbing news, particularly at the time of bereavement. This verse helps to console the family about their loss, signifying that nothing really belongs to us, not even our own lives, but is a trust from God.

Solace is often found in religion through prayers and reciting the *Quran.* The concept of *sabr,* or accepting God's will and wisdom, may be difficult to adopt initially and may cause additional spiritual pain and conflict.

Family and friends will often be around to offer solace and support. Any type of professional counselling will need to incorporate an Islamic understanding in order to be completely effective, as much of the anxiety and questions will be concerning one's relationship with God and understanding of the afterlife.

The funeral

The body undergoes a ritual washing (*ghusl*) by relatives of the same gender, although females can give a *ghusl* to a baby boy. The body is treated with great respect and gentleness through to burial. During washing it is not exposed but washed whilst a sheet is held in place to preserve the person's dignity. It is washed in a similar way to the ritual ablution and scented. It is then wrapped in a scented white sheet – camphor is usually used for this purpose. A non-Muslim can perform the ritual washing if no Muslims are available. After preparation, the body will be taken to the home or mosque. It will usually not be left on its own, but a vigil of prayers will be kept until the burial.

The funeral is a collective community duty. The more people at a funeral the more reward for the deceased. One does not have to have known the deceased, or be invited to a funeral; in fact it is a meritorious act to pray a funeral prayer. There is no official dress code. Some cultures may prefer to wear white or black; simple dress style is often implemented. The body will be buried in a Muslim graveyard. Babies can be buried in a multiple grave with others, even of non-Muslim parents, as all children are considered innocent and pure. Burial should take place as soon as practically possible. This so that the soul can go to rest and to preserve the appearance of the body. Embalming is discouraged. Any delay in burial may cause great distress. Muslims are always buried, never cremated. This is because of the belief in respecting the body as if it was alive. The body will be carefully looked after before burial.

Continuing bonds

Death does not end the relationship. Rewards of charitable acts, good actions and prayers can be sent as gifts to the departed soul. Often there are remembrances on the anniversary and set periods after death in the form of prayers, charity and good works. There can be communication through dreams and there is hope of being together in the hereafter.

A CONDOLENCE LETTER SENT BY THE PROPHET MUHAMMAD TO A COMPANION M'UAD

In the name of Allah the compassionate the Merciful. May peace be on you! I praise Allah the One. May Allah add to your recompense and calm your sad heart and give you endurance to thank him. As a matter of fact, our lives, our kith and kin and our property are merely a trust temporarily reposed in us from amongst the gifts of Allah. He benefits His servants by it till He likes and when the fixed time comes He takes it back. The duty of a man is to thank Allah, when He bestows on him a blessing and when He takes it back, he should endure it with patience. Your son was a good trust of Allah. He kept you blessed with him, till he liked. And when he desired He took him away from you. In return for a great recompense, provided you keep yourself content with Allah's will.

Oh M'uad if you show impatience you will lose your recompense and reward with Allah. If you get to know how much return and recompense has been granted to you for it, then this loss will appear very meagre in your eyes.

The promise which Allah has made with the people who endure misfortune and pain with patience shall be fully fulfilled in the life to come. The promise of Allah should reduce your grief. Whatever is destined to take place must occur.

Peace be there

Allah's Prophet, Muhammad

Key festivals

Mawlib-un-Nabi: The Prophet's birthday.

Ramadan: A month of fasting and self-discipline.

Eid-ul-Fitr: Celebrating the end of Ramadan.

Hajj: Pilgrimage to Makkah, one of the Five Pillars of Islam.

Lailat-ul-Barat: Means 'night of forgiveness' and takes place two weeks before the beginning of Ramadan.

Eid-ul-Adha: 'Big Eid' marks the end of Hajj and commemorates the story of Ibrahim's willingness to sacrifice his son.

There may be some discrepancies of a day either way for all of the festivals as Islam uses the lunar calendar, which means that dates become earlier by approximately ten days each year. The method of moon sighting varies, so you may find Muslims celebrating the festivals on different days. Eids are great family occasions and include fine food, clothes, thanksgiving presents and charity. These festivals could bring extra pain and sadness for those with a child in an end-of-life situation.

Celebrating Ramadan and Eid-ul-Fitr

Ramadan is celebrated in the ninth month of the Muslim calendar when the full moon is seen in the sky, and is often associated with the practice of fasting between sunrise and sunset. Fasting is about learning self-discipline and encouraging generosity as one remembers those who have little food. Eid-ul-Fitr is the celebration of the end of Ramadan and is a time of forgiveness and making amends, an occasion to give gifts to children and spend time with family and friends, and to give money to charity. Ways of celebrating include decorating crescent and star symbols linking this to the importance of paying attention to the moon; making biscuits or decorating biscuits to celebrate the end of Ramadan and fasting; playing pass the parcel with small gifts; and perhaps facts about Ramadan and Eid to emphasize the giving aspect; making Eid cards; decorating hands with *mhendi* (henna) patterns. In a hospital context it is particularly important to help families celebrate Eid as they are unable to join their family and friends in doing this.

Further reading

Hussain, Z. (2010) *A Gift for the Bereaved Parent.* London: Ta-Ha Publishing.
Hussain, Z. (2013) *Caring for the Muslim Child in Hospital.* Birmingham: Red Balloon Resources.

Hussain, Z. (2013) *Support for Muslim families who Have Been Told their Child is Incurable*. Birmingham: Red Balloon Resources.

Hussain, Z. (2013) *We Will Meet Again in Jannah*. London: Ta-Ha Publishing.

Notes

1   University of Granada (2011) 'Eating disorders and body dissatisfaction is double in Muslim teenagers than in Christian, Spanish study finds.' *Science Daily*, 8 March. Available at www.sciencedaily.com/releases/2011/03/110308084751.htm, accessed on 11 February 2014.

2   Bukhari is one of the collectors of Ahadith (recorded sayings and practice of the Prophet Muhammad). *Sahih Al-Bukhari*, tr. Dr Muhammad Muhsin Khan (1986). Lahore: Kazi Publications.

3   Blood is drawn by vacuum from small skin incisions at different points on the body for therapeutic purposes.

4   Banerjee, A.T., Watt, L., Gulati, S., Sung, L. *et al.* (2011) 'Cultural beliefs and coping strategies related to childhood cancer.' *Journal of Pediatric Oncology Nursing 28*, 3, 169–178.

7

CARE OF A SIKH CHILD AND FAMILY

Madeleine Parkes with
Parkash Sohal and Surinder Sidhu[1]

Introduction to Sikhism

Sikh means 'learner' or 'seeker of truth'. Sikhism was founded in 1469 in Punjab, North India, by Guru Nanak Dev Ji, and is both a religion and a way of life for many of its people. It is a philosophy to live by and focuses strongly on ethical conduct and earthly considerations, whilst always remembering God and the Gurus. Sikhs believe in one God and have a commitment to equality, justice and helping others. There are 25 million Sikhs around the world, with approximately 80 per cent of these residing in India.

21ST-CENTURY SIKHISM IN AUSTRALIA

Sikhs enter the 21st century with a great deal of optimism. They were part of the Commonwealth Centennial celebrations in 2001. They have won the respect of many European Australians who have assisted them in integrating into Australian society. The turban is a statement of their religious identity. Since the bombing of the World Trade Centre in the USA in 2001, they have faced harassment and physical abuse due to mistaken identity issues but have handled these as calmly as possible. The internal mix of the community is enabling them to involve themselves in various spheres of activity in Australian life.[2]

All Sikhs follow the same teachings of the Ten Gurus, although it would be incorrect to refer to 'the Sikh community' as one large homogenous group, as many Sikh communities are made up of groups of different people. The information provided below on culture, religion and spirituality should be taken as a starting point, from where you can be made aware of some of the differences you may encounter. However, the golden rule always applies, no matter how much factual knowledge you have read – *ask, don't assume*.

Beliefs and rituals

The founding Guru of Sikhism preached a message of love and understanding. The message of 'Ek Onkar' means, 'We are all one, created by the one creator of all creation.' Sikhism emphasizes the importance of community or brotherhood for Sikhs. After baptism (see below) Sikhs can usually be recognized because they wear five symbols that identify them as part of the Sikh brotherhood. These are the 5Ks:

1. *Kesh*: Hair is seen as a God-given gift and will not be cut. Hair on the head will be kept tidy by wearing a turban or headscarf, and this is one of the key symbols of Sikh identity you may find a Sikh wearing.

2. *Kanga*: This comb keeps the hair clean and tidy. Sikhs must comb their hair twice a day and tie their turbans neatly out of respect.

3. *Kara*: This is a silver-coloured bracelet that is a reminder to refrain from bad deeds. A Sikh may wear this on the right wrist to make him or her think twice about the actions of their hands.

4. *Kirpan*: This small sword is kept on the person. It is not used as a weapon, as Sikhism advocates peace and compassion. It is a symbol of courage and justice and serves as a reminder to fight against oppression and fight to preserve truth.

5. *Kachehra*: These are shorts or undergarments that are a reminder of chastity and self-control over human vices.

Concept of worship in Sikhism

The holy book of the Sikhs is called the *Guru Granth Sahib* and is written in *Gurmukhi*, a script commonly used to express the Punjabi language. It contains words and hymns and is considered sacred in and of itself – a living Guru. In the *gurdwara*, or Sikh temple, the main object of worship is a copy of this sacred book and it is raised up on a small table. Worshippers sit on the floor in front of it. Sikh priests, known as *granthi*, may be paid or unpaid and will conduct funerals, weddings and lead the prayers and singing in the *gurdwara*. The *Guru Granth Sahib* is read almost continuously: alternatively, there will usually be a recording playing or people will sing hymns. *Gurdwara* means 'gate of the Guru' and is usually open all day to receive people for prayers and worship. The first prayers are offered by Sikh families very early in the morning, with evening prayers and prayers before sleep also being offered later in the day. In the *gurdwara*, between prayer times, people can come and go freely and stay as long as they wish. Throughout this time the *Granth* is being read.

When worship occurs in a congregation (*sadh sangat*) the members will say prayers, sing hymns (*gurbani*) and listen to a teaching. Often this is followed by a free communal meal (*langar*) where everyone is invited to share food. Most Sikhs will have a copy of the prayer book known as the *Nitnem Banis* which means 'daily practice'. It contains sacred prayers to be recited regularly. In the home it is common practice to have a picture of a Guru displayed as a reminder of the faith.

Names and greetings

Many Sikhs in the West will offer a handshake in greeting. The traditional way of greeting is with folded hands and a small bow to the other person. This is especially the case when greeting a person of the opposite sex. The traditional Sikh greeting is *Sat Sri Akal* meaning God is the Truth. Sikh males or females who have family ties or are close to one another may embrace one another. Sikhs do not exchange a kiss on the cheek. Sometimes, older members of the family may place the palm of their hand on the head of a child or young adult, which symbolizes love and affection.

Popular surnames include Singh, meaning 'lion' (for men) and Kaur meaning 'princess' (for women). This surname may indicate the family are dedicated Sikhs, but as always, confirm this before assuming. Many Sikh families now also choose to add an additional surname to ensure they can be identified amongst the many Singhs and Kaurs. This may be a family name or the name of the village from which the family originates.

Family life

Sikhism teaches that God is to be found in daily life. The founders of Sikhism rejected monasticism and isolation, emphasizing active participation in daily life. Sikhs are encouraged to live by three key rules. First, they must meditate and focus on God. Second, they must share with others and third, they must earn their livelihood by honest means.

Sikhism does not specify that marriage should be arranged; rather, this practice is influenced by culture not religion. Arranged marriage is still a prevalent practice and some people in the West have misinformed views of this practice. Some Sikh couples will have had their marriage arranged by their families, with mutual agreement between all four parties involved. Sikhs are permitted to have only one husband or one wife. As marriage is seen as sacred, adultery is forbidden and divorce uncommon, although increasing in the West.

THE ROLE OF WOMEN IN FAMILY LIFE

Sikhism emphasizes total equality between man and woman, as well as all races. Women can participate in any religious function and lead the congregation.

The Guru said that God made mothers because he doesn't have enough time for us. He also said, 'The true path to God does not mean a renunciation of the world but through living the life of a householder, earning an honest living and avoiding temptation and sin', which emphasizes the role of family life for everyone.

The historical caste system, which originated in India, still has influence amongst some Sikh families, although this is changing. There are now many Sikh couples who are from different 'castes' that have married and raised families. The restrictions the caste system brings are declining.

Sikhs can use contraception, and assisted reproductive technologies are permitted. However, abortion is not permitted unless there is a serious threat to the mother's life. For a Sikh, the point at which a baby is conceived represents the soul's entry into the world.

Sikh families often live as a large extended group and not a nuclear family. It may be that three of four generations are living in the same household, or that extended family members all live near each other. For this reason family relationships may be large and complex.

Languages

The likely languages spoken by Sikhs include Punjabi and Hindi. The older generation in an immigrant family may speak little or no English. Young adults and children who are second, third or fourth generation immigrants may speak little or no Punjabi or Hindi.

Stories and attitudes to children

It is believed that children are a gift of God. Children in a Sikh household are usually active in their faith from the beginning, so, for example, a six-year-old might have a very good understanding of the faith. Parents will involve children in rituals to imbibe traditional Sikh values – to respect parents, demonstrate good behaviour, be polite, listen properly, answer with respect and show respect for elders. A common understanding is that if a person has parents at home then the home is sacred and full of blessings. Punjabi classes for children are usually available in the *gurdwara*.

A child may be 'baptized' into Sikhism when the child has a fair understanding of the faith. At this point they would wear a turban, which is understood to be a special gift which brings with it responsibility. For this ceremony they would attend the *gurdwara* for formal prayer, undertake a ritual bath and be presented with the five symbols of belonging to the Sikh brotherhood (more commonly known as the 5Ks – see above). Only baptized children wear the 5Ks, although some children may wear the steel bangle because they want to and as a sense of identity. Some younger children may not be able to tie the turban and may wear a *patka* instead, which is a small head covering. This is usually worn up until the age of about 11 when a child can learn to tie a turban.

The story of the youngest Guru

At the age of five, Guru Har Krishan Sahib Ji became the eighth Guru of the Sikhs (of ten). His wisdom and spiritual insights were revered, compared to the image of 'the early morning sun, looks small in size, but its light is everywhere'. Guru Har Krishan was taken suddenly ill with fever, which became smallpox. The Guru's mother, Mata Sulakkhani, became very sad. She said, 'Son, you are the dispeller of the world's sorrows and sufferings. Your very sight removes the ailments of others. Why do you lie sick now?' Guru Har Krishan replied, 'He who has taken this mortal frame must go through sickness and disease. Both happiness and suffering are part of life. What is ordained must happen. This is what Guru Nanak taught. Whatever He does is His order. One must walk in the light of His command.'

His mother, with tears in her eyes, said 'How shall I live without thee, son? I was blessed when I came into this family married to the late Guru. I was blessed when you were born. Now I am cast into a bottomless ocean of sorrow. Who would be my rescuer? How does a fish live separated from water?' 'The body is perishable,' said Guru Har Krishan. 'As you learn to have faith in God's Will, you will attain to realms sorrowless. Eternal peace will be yours.' Guru Har Krishan in 1664 at the age of 8.[3]

Care of Sikh patients and their families in hospital

There is a belief that God looks after you in a congregation, and although you can pray anywhere, there are extra blessings (*sangat*) in a congregation. For many families and children the *gurdwara* is an important part of daily life. Children who are ill are still welcomed in a *gurdwara*, and although they are religiously exempt from religious duties they will probably wish to go more frequently.

There is a good chance that older generations of the same family will be looking after children in hospital. Many Sikhs, especially of an older generation, have an active temple life and visit the *gurdwara* regularly – sometimes daily or several times a day. As this may be their main source of both spiritual and social life, this may be missed in hospital and it would be important to make the family aware of any prayer space or religious provision in the hospital. Sikh chaplaincy could help with the carer's isolation and own wellbeing.

Food and prohibited products

Sikhism emphasizes that food should be eaten in a simple and nutritious form. Some Sikhs will choose to be vegetarian or restrict meat from their diets for different reasons, including cultural and health reasons. Some Sikhs will understand the teaching to live in harmony with the world to include not eating meat. The original teachings on this issue are complex and the decision is down to the individual. However, many Sikhs believe it is mandatory to be vegetarian once baptized and it is very important for those Sikhs not to have any meat, fish or egg products. Even inadvertent consumption would be considered a major sin by some Sikhs and they would need to go through the baptism ceremony again and ask for forgiveness.

Sikh scriptures forbid the eating of meat killed in ways that other religions require. This would include meat killed in the Muslim tradition (*halal*) and Jewish tradition (*kosher*). It is therefore very important to clarify the child's faith before assuming they need a particular type of religious food as the provision of the incorrect food could cause significant offence. The consumption of tobacco, alcohol or other intoxicants is forbidden on the grounds of fitness and health. However, some people may partake of these substances. Food served at the *gurdwara* will always be vegetarian to avoid offence and to meet the range of dietary requirements of its many visitors. Some Sikhs will practise the principle of *joodh*, which means that utensils that have been used to serve prohibited food will not be used. After these items have been washed they are acceptable to most Sikhs. However, some baptized Sikhs would prefer separate utensils to be used for the preparation of vegetarian and non-vegetarian food if at all possible.

Modesty and hygiene

This will be age specific but many children will have concerns about modesty, like any other child. Some Sikh children will adhere to the principle of letting hair grow. However, it has been noted that in modern Sikhism some young Sikhs are less concerned with this principle. For teenagers, both male and female, who are strong adherents to the faith, facial hair is also not shaved or trimmed. Many Sikhs will be accustomed to removing their shoes and washing their hands, and sometimes their feet, prior to prayer or entering a place of worship.

Taboos

Taboos and stigma are still big problems amongst Sikhs, specifically around sexuality, mental illness and abuse. There is huge community pressure, the risk of getting a 'bad' name and the stigma of speaking out. Children may also suffer as they may be forbidden to talk.

Sexuality is not openly discussed, which may create problems within the family or wider community. It is seen as entertainment in India, where men dress in clothing of the other gender as part of a joke. Sexuality is not really talked about amongst Sikhs, and there are no explicit teachings about homosexuality in the *Guru Granth Sahib*. However, there is a focus on married life between a man and a woman, so many Sikhs see this as implying that homosexuality is forbidden. Other Sikhs may see the absence of teachings around this to mean that it is not an issue. Cultural influences on these opinions will be great, and some families will choose to ignore issues of sexuality.

Alcohol and drug taking are strongly discouraged in Sikhism, so a child or teenager who has been using these substances may cause disbelief or disgust in the family. Suicide is a taboo subject in most Sikh families due to the stigma from some members of the community.

By the bedside

It is unlikely that Sikh scriptures will be found by the bedside of a child in hospital. The scriptures are considered sacred in themselves. However, some families may have a copy, wrapped in a cloth or enclosed in a case, which may be placed by the bedside. These portable copies may have a cover with a special message to remind the user to handle it with respect and reverence. Great respect should be shown to this book. It should not be touched unless you have asked permission and have washed your hands. Other items should not be placed on top of it. Sometimes the case or covering of the book will indicate that within are holy scriptures and it should be handled with care.

The child or teenager could be wearing a steel bangle from a very young age. The steel bangle, worn by many Sikhs, should not be removed. Usually there is an alternative way to conduct medical procedures without removing the bangle, such as by taping it up. Respect the 5Ks on the body and any head covering, and do not remove the 5Ks unless absolutely necessary, explaining why they need to be removed. Always ask permission before doing so. There may also be pictures of a Guru, which could indicate faith during struggle, hope and safety. It could also be an important part of the child and family's identity and may be on display at the bedside as an indicator of belonging, and the images will be shown respect and care. The child may be wearing a *Khanda* necklace, which would indicate their faith. The *Khanda* refers to both the 'brotherhood' of Sikhism and the symbol that is often used in conjunction with the faith. It may be obvious that the child or teenager in the bed space follows the Sikh faith as they may have long, uncut hair tied in a knot, or under a *patka* or turban. Sikhs do not believe in fasting or pilgrimage, and therefore these are not religious needs for a Sikh family.

Although the child, siblings and perhaps parents will speak and understand English, it is likely that older generations will not. Even parents who have a good level of English may find medical terminology difficult to understand, as they may not have heard it before and the concepts may not be easily translatable. A translator may be needed; the likely languages spoken by Sikhs include Punjabi and Hindi. Every effort should be made to use a professional translator, not a family member of the patient. Where practical a Sikh chaplain may be able to offer translation skills. If using a family member to translate, be very mindful that they are hearing the news you are telling them for the first time and may not fully understand what is being said. If they do understand they may not be able to find the most accurate words to translate the information

A CHAPLAIN'S VIEW

I visited a family with a newborn daughter. Her parents were very anxious and concerned all day and all night. I spent a lot of time with them, explaining who and what was available in the hospital – hospitals can be a bewildering place for families in distress. I also offered them my contact details with an invitation to call on me in times of worry or distress. I got to know the family well enough to offer prayers before and after the little girl's operation. It was important for me to be a consistent presence – I saw them every few days and offered as much time as possible, being a source of comfort.

into – this is particularly true for unfamiliar medical terminology or concepts – and they should be invited to clarify their understanding with you.

It is important to respect times of prayer and a praying patient and their family should not be interrupted.

Age-specific considerations

Babies and infants

Be aware that some Sikhs will not want to feed their babies or infants meat or eggs. Check the ingredients in baby food before supplying it. Breast-feeding is encouraged in Sikhism but is down to personal choice. Baby naming ceremonies are conducted, but there is no specific length of time after birth in which this has to be completed. The baby will be presented to the *Guru Granth Sahib*, and various prayers and hymns will be said and sung. Male infants are not circumcized.

Children

Small pieces of scripture or a book of scripture may be near the bedside. This will be wrapped in cloth and carefully looked after. Prayer beads might be present around the wrist. Various websites are designed for Sikh children to find out more about their faith, and Sikhism encourages reflecting and thinking on beliefs as well as exploring different religions out of interest, without compromising one's own.

Even young children may be wearing the 5Ks. These items should not be removed unless absolutely necessary and with consent; alternatives to removing them should always be explored. If they are removed they might then be stored under the pillow or looked after by the family. If a child on the ward is displaying the 5Ks this indicates how important Sikhism is to them. As part of the 5Ks, any hair on the body must not be cut.

Teenagers

A turban or other head covering may be worn as a sign of spiritual maturity. It is considered a sacred gift, and with it comes the responsibility of following the Sikh path. There are many different types of head coverings across many different faiths, so you should confirm that the head covering indicates a Sikh child or family before assuming so. Although younger children can choose to commit to Sikhism it might be more difficult for teenagers and young adults to practise their faith in hospital due to the seriousness with which they practise their faith. Understand the importance of the decision they have made to become a baptized Sikh. A teenage Sikh might struggle to be devout and conform to the requirements of their faith whilst in hospital.

Prayers and hymns may be recorded on electronic devices and could be an important way for a young adult Sikh to practise their faith. It would be vitally important to consult the teenage patient prior to shaving or removing hair from any part of their body, including facial and pubic hair. This applies to both male and female patients and relates to the Sikh mandate not to shave or remove hair as it is a symbol of God's creation. For teenage women, hirsutism or excessive hair growth on the face, neck, chest and back can be difficult to cope with, especially in a Western society that has cultural expectations of shaving 'unwanted' hair. There are many teenage Sikh women who have proudly embraced their facial hair despite potential and actual stigma. Sometimes for a Sikh child or teenager they will be torn between being independent and in control of their own wishes and respecting the adults around them, which is an important value taught from a young age.

Working with the family

Respect is important both culturally and spiritually. Use respectful terms to address adult family members and be wary of making eye contact and smiling with elderly adult members of the family as this can be culturally inappropriate – watch for clues, such as aversion of eyes. Take a very sensitive and gentle approach.

Any patient and their family would prefer staff to ask them about their faith and religious practices rather than assume and cause offence. *Sat Sri Akal* is the traditional Sikh greeting, and a Sikh family would be delighted to hear staff greet them in this way as it acknowledges their faith and identity. This should only be attempted when staff have established that the family are practising Sikhs. There are likely to be many visitors to the child and carers in hospital. This will need to be managed sensitively by ward staff and accommodated where possible. If there is a side room or quiet room where the family can gather this would be appreciated. The family should also be made aware of any available prayer space or religious provision in the hospital.

Conducive environment

Sikhs would appreciate symbols and items from other religions to be removed from their child's bed space. Sikhs are very respectful of other world faiths; however, they would prefer not to see other symbols as they may be considered idol worship, which is forbidden. An image of the Guru or the symbol of the *Khanda* is permissible. Sikhs will wear head coverings and remove their shoes in special places such as the temple or places that are considered sacred or important.

Offence would be caused if a Sikh was mistaken for a Muslim (or vice versa). There might be some confusion around headgear and food, and every effort should be made to ask, not assume. Sadly, many Sikhs, as well as many Muslims, are victims of abuse from people who label them all as 'terrorists' through lack of awareness and understanding. Both faiths teach peace. Symbols of the faiths worn by Muslims and Sikhs are different and most people, even with a small amount of religious awareness and sensitivity, would recognize this.

Water is seen as purifying and calming, and may be sprinkled around important religious items or the bed in order to ensure the area around it is spiritually pure.

Views of suffering

Some families will have no knowledge of some illnesses, as the illness is not known in their community or there is lack of education around it. A common question is, 'Why is this happening to us?' or 'Why me?' We can all acknowledge that this is an extremely difficult question to answer, and families and patients may look towards their religious and spiritual understanding of illness and suffering to explain this. A Sikh family may be encouraged by the chaplain to think about the present and future, focusing on caring and providing comfort for the child. The family may have some medical understanding but will often ascribe suffering and illness to bad deeds done in the past. A

Sikh chaplain may encourage prayer in order to lessen the impact of these deeds and promote healing. A patient and their family will be encouraged to think positively; they may also be sprinkled with holy water and encouraged to meditate on qualities of God. Some Sikh families may have their beliefs challenged and lose faith in God. Some Sikhs may have cultural practices that they adhere to but have little or no religious belief. Families should be reassured that they have done nothing wrong, and that the body, health and illness are all given by God. God's will plays an important part in Sikh belief and although this may be hard to believe it can be a comfort as it removes blame from the family. There may not always be an answer but illness and suffering are not a punishment.

Breaking bad news is never easy. Sikhs will be encouraged to pray and to believe that God will heal if that is His will. Some families will be very distressed if the issue of death and bereavement are raised as they may not wish to think of this and may still hope God will heal. The illness of a girl or young woman can cause more concern amongst families. This is because girls can be considered important to extend the family and to form a new household. This may have an impact on family relations if a female child dies.

EXPLAINING SUFFERING – A CHAPLAIN'S VIEW

It is very common for people to explain suffering as a result of past bad deeds. I saw a toddler who was admitted to hospital with severe burns as a result of a cup of tea. When I went to the burns unit the mother kept saying it was her fault and that she shouldn't have put the cup there. I said to her, 'You didn't want your child to be burnt. If you keep blaming yourself you won't be able to look after him… Guru said God is forgiving and compassionate, Guru said that God made mothers because he doesn't have enough time for us, so we offer love and care in his place.'

Attitudes to medical care

Understanding illness and disease

Some physical illnesses have more stigma and misunderstanding attached to them than others. For example, some people believe that cancer is contagious and therefore the family may keep a child's diagnosis secret from the wider community. Many Sikhs are called to help those who are suffering. However, out of curiosity and lack of knowledge, some will come to see how the illness looks in the child, or how the child copes in a wheelchair or with no hair. A common explanation for illness is that someone, either the child or immediate family member, has done something bad in a past life and they are now experiencing the effects in this life. For this reason, suffering is seen to be hereditary from previous lives. Prayers will be said for the child at temple or at home. The family may request that a continuous reading of the *Granth*, known as *Akhand Path*, which takes around 48 hours, can be dedicated to the ill child and their family.

ATTITUDES TO MEDICAL CARE

Almost all forms of medical treatment are permitted for Sikhs, and indeed medical treatment to treat illnesses is encouraged by the faith. Sikhism values the sciences and the knowledge of healthcare practitioners, and Sikhs are not prohibited from using any medical procedures. However, cutting any hair is considered to be disrespectful; some patients resist shaving the hair on the body before an operation or for medical investigation. (UK Sikh Healthcare Chaplaincy Group)[4]

Understanding mental illness

There is a real lack of understanding about mental illness within Sikh communities. Socially and culturally these conditions are stigmatized, mainly because of the belief in the unlikelihood of the child finding a marriage partner and the status of the family. There may be a suspicion about mental illness, which can cause tension. Some people will believe that it is the parents' fault that a child or teenager has a mental health problem and some members of the community will suspect that the rest of the family also has problems. This can impact the status of the family in the community and affect future relationships. There is a good chance the family won't want to tell anyone in the community and they may therefore have a lack of community support.

In young people juggling a Western and a Sikh culture and identity, mental illness can be overlooked by families. Young people may have a lot more awareness, language and knowledge. Many families may focus on the causes not solutions of mental health problems. There are some words describing mental illness that do not translate into Punjabi, and the label 'mad' (*pagal*) is a very bad label to have and can deeply affect relationships. Some people may ascribe superstitious beliefs to the causes of illness. In some South Asian cultures there is a superstitious notion of 'the evil eye' causing illness, including mental illness, as well as *jadu-tona* (black magic) and *bhuta preta* (malevolent ghosts or spirits of people who have died). These are cultural not religious beliefs and the Sikh chaplain will be able to help a family understand this better. Historically, the Sikh Gurus rejected suicide because of the belief that we haven't got the right to give or take life. Birth and death are at the mercy of God. The reaction to a suicide would depend on how good the family are at putting themselves in the person's shoes. Sikh chaplains would like to help the family of a person who has committed suicide and would like to support a shift in the mindset of the person who has attempted suicide.

Pain management

A *shabaad* is a sacred song based on Sikh scripture. It can be sung at any time, although for a child and family in hospital there may be specific hymns sung. *Shabaads* do not require to be understood in order for the grace imparted from them to have an effect. Therefore, they can be used for children of all ages and cognitive abilities.

Meditation is seen as a solution to mental illness. Meditation on God specifically, in order to relax the body and mind, is a popular response to mental health problems. *Naam Simram* is a meditation practice that focuses on the loving remembrance of God – a meditation practice that requires not ritual but just the person to calm the mind and remember the supreme soul. It also helps the patient to focus on something other than him- or herself, which can be helpful.

A shabaad for healing: *Gourree Mehalaa 5* – Composed in Measure Gauree, by Fifth Guru

> One who would stand with me from the start, midway and to the end.
> My mind longs for such a Friend,
> The Lord's Love goes ever with us.

The Perfect Merciful Master cherishes all.
He shall perish not, and shall never abandon me.
Wherever I look, there I see Him pervading.
Beautiful, All-knowing, and most Clever, is the Giver of life.

God is Brother, Son, Father and Mother.
He is the Support of my life breath; He is my Wealth.
Abiding within my heart, The Lord inspires me to enshrine love for
    Him.
The noose of Maya is cut away by the Lord of the World.

Beholding me with His blessed gracious glance He has made me
    His own.
By ever remembering Him in contemplation are all diseases healed.

By focusing on His Feet, are all comforts enjoyed.
The Perfect Omnipresent Lord is ever fresh and ever young.
Within and without is the Lord with me, as my Protector.
Says Nanak, the Lord, God is realized.
Blessed with all of the Name's treasure is the devotee.[5]

Traditional healing and medicine

Belief in 'hot' and 'cold' foods

Certain foods are believed to have a 'cooling' or 'heating' effect on
the function of various organs of the body. The concept is divorced
from the actual temperature of food or even how spicy the food is,
but is about the effect it has on the body. 'Hot' foods, such as lentils,
aubergines and eggs, are thought to increase physical and emotional
activity, and 'cold' foods, such as milk, white sugar, fruits and cereals
have a calming effect. Such customs as a glass of water/metal under a
baby's cot/black string tied around a baby's wrist or ankle are more
cultural than religious, and may be passed through generations. There
may be a belief that the baby may be vulnerable to evil spirits and
these items offer protection.[6]

Talking therapy

Counselling is not hugely popular in South Asian communities but its popularity is increasing and for a Sikh there is a Sikh model of spiritual counselling available. The basis of this is that one should be God centred (*gurmukh*) not self-centred (*manmukh*), which could be a useful tool in talking therapy with a Sikh patient.

Understanding death

Sikhs believe that life and death is like a map that God has laid out for you. God's will, or *hukam*, is a strong belief in Sikhism. God is both compassionate and a mystery, and the Gurus become a focus in Sikh religious practice because they make God's compassion and wisdom real and relatable. Sikhs may turn to the teachings of the Gurus to understand death. Accepting the will of God in the hardest circumstances is a great human achievement. However, although Sikhism teaches that God's will pervades life and death this is not always easy to accept when a child dies. It may relieve some of the guilt or blame people may ascribe to the death. With regard to the belief in *karma* and reincarnation, there may be a comforting belief that as humans who are subject to reaping what we sow, we work out the results of this on earth. Therefore, some souls only need to be in human form briefly – a young child. This can be comforting, but also still difficult.

Preparing for death

Life support is permitted in Sikhism. However, the decision still needs to be made according to the family's wishes, and they would appreciate being told the realities of recovery and likely quality of life before making the decision. Sikh families with a strong faith will continue to live with the hope of a miracle even when the condition is terminal. Although family members would appreciate knowing the realities of the approaching death, they may choose not to share this news with the wider family in order to be seen to be keeping a positive attitude.

When a child is approaching death:

- Last prayers (*ardass*) are read. A local faith leader or a Sikh chaplain is likely to be requested.

- Prayers must be by the bedside, with the family around.

- Parents may sprinkle holy water on the body or if possible they may encourage the child to sip it, or at least have some placed on their tongue. The family might have holy water with them but usually it can be provided by the Sikh chaplain.

- The child should be kept as comfortable as possible, and the family should have access to parts of the *Guru Granth Sahib*.

Immediately after death:

- Sikhs console themselves by reciting their sacred hymns. No other rites are required.

- Wailing and strong expressions of grief are discouraged, due to the belief that death is God's will and the soul has moved on.

- The 5Ks must be kept intact, even when washing the body.

- Hands should be placed by the side, and the usual last offices can be performed by the nursing staff.

- The family is responsible for all religious ceremonies and rites associated with death and may want to wash the body themselves.

- Hair is considered sacred, and it is particularly important *not* to offer a lock of hair from the child's head for remembrance purposes.

- The body should be wrapped in a clean white cloth.

WHEN RELIGIOUS CARE DOESN'T GO WELL…

Prayer is very powerful for many Sikhs, and we can say lots of different prayers depending on the circumstances we face. However, if a patient dies, some people might believe that we have not said enough prayers and may lose faith or feel that there was more they could have done.

Organ donation and post-mortem

There are no religious objections to organ donation. It may be encouraged as an act of service to humanity, or *seva*, which is a fundamental concept in Sikhism. There may, however, be some cultural concerns that organ donation means that the person's spirit will not leave the body at the end of their life or that somehow a part of their body will live forever. From a religious perspective post-mortem is accepted, although there may be cultural or personal resistance.

Hospice care

There is nothing religious to say about hospice care. It is a family decision, but there will be a common understanding that it's the family's responsibility and the best care would be given by family at home. There is a fear that people in the community will start talking and perhaps cast judgements about the parents not being able to look after their own child. Hospices are not commonly known amongst Sikhs and people may not realize that they are places for palliative and end-of-life care – this should be explained carefully and the family should be assured that their child will be taken very good care of. Specific information will be most important.

Caring for the family after the death of their child

A Sikh religious leader can be called to visit the bereaved family at home, as well as the family making visits to *gurdwara*. The local community may be able to offer practical, emotional and even financial help.

The focus should be on supporting the parents. Blaming the parents, especially the mother, can be attributed by others (due to cultural conditioning), which goes against principles of Sikhism. God's will is a great comfort. It is considered a great spiritual achievement to accept the will of God, as it is known that faith is easy when things are easy. Please

CONDOLENCES

It is appropriate to call and express care and love for the deceased. However, it is important to focus on the positives of the person's life and minimize the sadness and loss as much as is possible. Flowers, gifts and contributions to charity in the person's name are welcomed but not necessary.

be wary of offering physical touch as a comfort to a grieving family, as this may not be culturally appropriate. Be led by the family.

The funeral

It is preferable that the body is released with minimal delay. Ideally the child should be cremated within 11 days of death, although some religious sources suggest 24 hours. The body will be removed to the funeral home for quick cremation, unless the family are waiting for other relatives to arrive.

The funeral ceremony is *antam sanska* (final rites). Although everything should be done within 11 days, if family members are travelling from abroad to attend the funeral this may take longer. Arrangements may be made to have a full reading of the *Guru Granth Sahib* – this may be started at home or in the *gurdwara*, whichever is suggested by the priest. Usually it is completed on the day of cremation. On the last day, after cremation, the *Sadh Ramkali* is read, which tells of the third Guru's death, the transitory nature of life and the acceptance of God's will. Although the funeral typically takes place within 11 days, some happen much sooner. In some Sikh communities, the body is taken to *gurdwara* to be blessed in front of the *Guru Granth Sahib*. In other communities the body is kept in a different room and prayers are said without the presence of the holy scriptures. All Sikhs are cremated. No memorials are erected and it is forbidden to commemorate anniversaries of the death. This is because of the Sikh belief that the body is simply a shell, and the soul will continue to live on in a different form.

The ashes are often scattered on a river or in the sea. Sometimes this involves a trip to India where ashes of previous family members were disposed of. Developed foetuses, stillborn babies, infants and children receive a full funeral in accordance with Sikh tradition – there is no difference due to age. The family may wish to name the baby if it was stillborn. The death rites of a child or adult person who has committed suicide will be conducted in the same way as any other death. The *Kirtan Sohila* prayer will often be said, which is a blessing for the departed soul. Family and elders may wear white during the period of mourning. The mourning period will be between two and five weeks, although it may be longer for a child.

> **DIFFERENCES BETWEEN ADULTS AND CHILDREN**
> Sikhism views death of a child as similar to that as an adult. There is to be no difference in the way in which the child is treated. This therefore involves cremation. There has been a practice in India of burying young children. However, in the west, this would mean that a grave allocated space would need to be purchased and this is not acceptable for Sikhs. Whilst this is practiced in many households in India, it does not have any grounding within the principles of the Sikh faith.[7]

Continuing bonds

This is not a recognized concept in Sikhism due to the belief that the child's soul has moved on, following the path of reincarnation. Remembering the child and performing acts in his or her memory are a different concept and are permitted. Some parents will choose to believe in continuing bonds as this may be a comfort, despite religious teachings.

Key festivals

Birthday of Guru Gobind Singh: Tenth and last Guru who instituted the 5Ks and the order of the Khasla.

Vaisaki: A festival marking the start of the Sikh New Year and commemorating the founding of the *Khalsa*, the Sikh 'brotherhood' or community, by the tenth Guru.

Martyrdom of Guru Arjan Dev ji: The fifth Sikh Guru and the first Sikh Martyr who compiled the Sikh scriptures into one book.

Diwali: The festival of lights, most popular Hindu/Sikh festival.

Birthday of Guru Nanak: Celebrating the birth of the founder of Sikhism. May be celebrated on the fixed date of 14 April.

Martyrdom of Guru Tegh Banabur: The ninth Sikh Guru honoured as champion of religious freedom.

Celebrating the martyrdom of Guru Arjan Dev ji

Guru Arjan Dev ji was the fifth Sikh Guru and the first Sikh Martyr. He put all of the past Gurus' writing into one book, laying the foundation for the Sikh holy scripture the *Guru Granth Sahib*. He laid the foundation of the Golden Temple in Amritsar. His martyrdom is sometimes celebrated by the sharing of cold drinks, so you could make smoothies or lemonade, for example. Another activity is to make a little book and encourage children to put their name and a picture inside and then answer questions like, 'Who inspires you and why?'

Further reading

Bakhshi, S.S. and Sohal, P.K. (2011) *Sikh Prayers for the Loss of a Child*. Birmingham: Red Balloon Resources.

Bakhshi, S.S. and Sohal, P.K. (2013) *Sikh Prayers for an Ill Child*. Birmingham: Red Balloon Resources.

Notes

1   With thanks to Dr Jaswant Singh Sohal for his input.
2   Adapted from Gurdarshan Singh Gill, *Sikhs in Australia*. Available at www.sikh.com.au/cgi-bin/index.cgi?page=27, accessed on 1 February 2014.
3   Adapted from Guru Har Krishan ji (1661–1664). Available at www.sikh-history.com/sikhhist/gurus/nanak8.html, accessed on 1 February 2014.
4   Singh, H. (2009) Caring for a Sikh Patient. London: Sikh Healthcare Chaplaincy Group. Available at www.covwarkpt.nhs.uk/aboutus/equality-and-diversity/Documents/Caring%20for%20a%20Sikh%20Patient.pdf, accessed on 18 January 2015.
5   http://sikhism.about.com/od/prayersforalloccasisions/a/Sikh-Hymn-For-Healing-Simar-Simar-Kattae-Sabh-Rog.htm
6   Adapted from Gatrad, R., Jhutti-Johal, J., Gill, P.S. and Sheikh, A. (2005) 'Sikh birth customs.' *Archives of Disease in Childhood 90*, 6, 560–563.
7   UK Sikh Healthcare Chaplaincy Group, *Guidance Note on Dealing with Bereavement in Sikh Families; Still Birth and Miscarriages*. Sikh Chaplaincy. Available at www.sikhchaplaincy.org.uk/~sikhchap/images/publications/guidance_note_on_dealing_with_bereavement_in_sikh_families.pdf, accessed on 1 December 2014.

8

SPIRITUAL CARE
Christmas in July for a Hindu Family

Claire Carson

Spiritual care is all about getting alongside people and listening to their stories, allowing space for the unpredictable and extraordinary. It involves creating a safe space in which people can be themselves, ask difficult questions, laugh, cry, talk or be silent, a respectful space which values all people of any religion or none. Of course, religious care is important too, especially for those people who identify with a specific religious tradition. Yet, if we only talk about religious care we may miss the point of what chaplaincy–spiritual care is all about and, indeed, why it is a valuable part of healthcare. Many people I see would not say they were 'religious', but they do value the opportunity to talk. For many patients, the experience of being ill, or experiencing a trauma of some kind, can turn their world upside down. It can challenge their identity: their perceptions of who they are and how they see their relationships. As Kelly states, 'The spiritual aspect of our human personhood is that element which seeks meaning and purpose in life. Such a dimension is not confined to persons of religious faith, but is part of what it is to be human.[1] I'm keen to remind people that although I'm an Anglican priest working as a hospital chaplain, my philosophy is that I'm here for everyone, regardless of whether they are religious or not.

Some people identify with a particular religion due to their culture. Therefore, some people may prefer to see only someone from their own tradition, but equally, others may feel comfortable talking to a chaplain of another faith, depending on their situation or experience. An example of this is the experience I had with a Hindu family whose son was dying on a children's ward. Although they were Hindu, they had links with the Church of England due to the fact that all of their children attended a Church of England school. These links formed a significant part of their lives and each year the family would celebrate Christmas.

Arvind's story

As part of my work, I regularly visit paediatric wards and work closely with the school bases. During one such visit in a busy hospital, one of the teachers called me to ask if I would visit a family on their ward. This family were struggling to come to terms with some bad news they had just been given: they had been made aware that their son Arvind was coming towards the end of his life. The teacher who made the referral had told the family about me and so I was able to approach them and introduce myself. The whole family – mum, dad, brother and sister – were present with Arvind. Although they were Hindu, they were happy to see an Anglican chaplain.

This was a close-knit family and they were determined to give Arvind the best care they could. They wanted to talk about what was happening and how they were feeling. They told me all about Arvind, his life and his illness: how Arvind had Duchenne Muscular Dystrophy, a serious condition which causes progressive muscle weakness. The onset of symptoms generally occur in early childhood, usually between the ages of three and five years. Arvind's swallowing muscles had become weak and he wasn't able to eat or drink. He then developed pneumonia, and at this point he was admitted into hospital. Arvind had been in and out of hospital many times that year, but this time his condition was so serious that he and his family were given the choice of whether he should spend his last months at home, in the hospital or in a hospice. They decided it was best to let Arvind stay where he was, especially as they knew the team of doctors and nurses, the massage therapist, the chaplain and the teachers. They felt settled there and, more importantly, felt that it was a safe place.

A teacher started to create a memory book with Arvind, and in the process asked him about what was important to him and what he liked doing. Through these conversations she discovered he loved Christmas. It was their family tradition to go to Midnight Mass every Christmas Eve and he was really sad that he was going to miss future festivities. Arvind really wanted to celebrate another Christmas before he died, and his family wanted more than anything to give him the chance to do this.

As I continued to visit the family regularly for general support, we began to discuss the idea of creating a Christmas celebration for Arvind in the last few weeks of his life. This was clearly important to all of the family as they longed so much to make Arvind's last few weeks special for him. Plans were put in place and I arranged for the hospital chapel to be decorated appropriately. Having talked with the family about how they would like the service to be, it became clear that they wanted to sing carols and have readings, and that they wanted it to end with a surprise visit from Santa! Celebrating Christmas in July was a surprise to all involved. Everyone, from the cleaners to the consultants, came together to help prepare this very special day. The hospital chapel was decked with more decorations than it usually is at Christmas! We even had a tree and lights. I put together a service book containing the carols and prayers. Some of the teachers agreed to act out the nativity from the book *Jesus' Christmas Party*.[2]

When the time came for the service to start, the nurses brought Arvind down to the chapel in his bed. He had been very unwell for a few days and we were all anxious as to whether he was going to be able to attend 'Christmas'. The chapel was full and you could see people trying extra hard not to cry as they celebrated with Arvind and his family. Leading the service was a very special privilege but I also found that holding everything together was exhausting. The depth of emotion in the room was tangible. There was a strange feeling all around. People walking past the chapel would stop, look for a moment and then realize what was going on. I don't think I met anyone who passed by that day who didn't have a tear in their eye. Arvind made it to the end of the carol service and even managed to smile many times from his bed. Then, to his surprise, Santa turned up with lots of gifts. It was a truly special day and one that had offered an opportunity for everyone to come together in mutual support.

After the Christmas celebration I continued to visit Arvind and his family as I had by this point built up a good relationship with everyone. Together we entered the next phase, which involved waiting and watching by Arvind's bedside as he deteriorated further. Conversations turned more towards what the family would like to happen when he came to the end of his life. As the ward Arvind was on very rarely had deaths, this raised several challenges. The family wanted to be able to give Arvind a bubble bath when he died and spend time with him in his room. They also requested that I accompany him to the mortuary and then meet them in the viewing room to see him. They were comfortable with me going with him because I had spent time at the ward and he knew me. They also wanted him to be wrapped in his favourite duvet cover rather than a hospital sheet. Through conversations, and collaboration with ward and mortuary staff, we were able to make sure the family's wishes were carried out.

The funeral

As Arvind was approaching the last few days of his life the family asked me if I would be able to conduct his funeral service. During this time I gently asked them about how they would like this service to be, and I worked with them to put the funeral service together. I assured them that I would be as flexible as possible and create with them a service that would reflect Arvind's life. We discussed what music and readings they wanted to include, as well as who they would like to talk about Arvind's life. To end the service it was decided that superhero balloons would be released. As Arvind's favourite colour was red, people were invited to wear bright colours to the funeral.

When Arvind died, I accompanied him, as requested, to the mortuary and arranged for regular family visits until his funeral, something which was very important for the family. The family requested an open coffin so people could see Arvind and say their farewells to him at home before the service and also during the service. They wanted rose petals to be sprinkled over him during the service at the crematorium as music played, before I did the commendation prayers. Rose petals symbolize life in the Hindu tradition and it was also a way for people to personally say goodbye to Arvind.

The service had a very spiritual feel without it being overtly religious. I used very open language; talking about an all-embracing, loving God, as well as themes of peace and hope. A funeral is always going to be difficult and painful for people, so I wanted to create an opportunity during which people could express their sadness and pain allowing them to come alongside each other and participate in this part of the journey for Arvind's family. I wanted it to have meaning and significance for the family, to be a creative, safe and respectful space, valuing who they are and their love for a very special son, brother and friend.

> Into the freedom of wind and sunshine, we let you go.
> Into the dance of the stars and the planets, we let you go.
> Into the wind's breath and the hands of the starmaker, we let you go.
> May you rest in peace and love now and always.[3]

Reflections

Working with Arvind and his family in the last few weeks of his life was a great privilege, and he was an inspiration to everyone who shared his journey. I felt incredibly welcomed into their lives as they shared with me their hopes and fears, their joys and sorrows. Occasionally they would remember times they had shared together as a family and tell me their stories. I was with them in their distress and sat with them through many difficult moments. I found words inadequate and was powerfully reminded of the significance of silence and the importance of just being with Arvind and his family in the pain and the mystery of life. There were no words that could be said, no answers that could be given; just silence and time passed together. It reminded me of the Janet Morley poem 'and you held me':

> And you held me and there were no words
> and there was no time and you held me
> and there was only wanting and
> Being held and being filled with wanting
> and I was nothing but letting go
> and being held
> and there were no words and there
> needed to be no words...[4]

Being there, being present was all I could do: offering them a space simply to be held – spiritually if not physically. Not running away from their pain and distress, but sitting with them. So often chaplaincy–spiritual care is misunderstood, sidelined and forgotten about. 'Who is the chaplain?' 'What do they do?' 'They're just for religious people!' Some people assume we're all very religious and all we do is pray with people.

My regular visits to Arvind provided me with a great opportunity to get to know the staff on the ward and deepen my relationship with them too. It was a chance to work closely with staff at all levels, really engaging in multidisciplinary teamwork. It also allowed me to explain my approach to chaplaincy–spiritual care. As a chaplain I frequently have an overview of what is going on and can use my role to bring people together. On this occasion I built up trust not only with Arvind's family but also with the staff, and I believe this enabled us to offer the best possible care. My role also allowed me to offer support to the staff, giving them space to talk about how they were feeling, as well as the challenges they were facing.

The nursing and medical staff were caring for many other children at the same time as Arvind. As mentioned above, the ward wasn't usually a place where children died. Indeed, the other children were all expected to recover and go home. The staff had to deal with caring for a dying child alongside recovering children, which was extremely difficult for them and required great skill, energy, dedication and commitment. I think it also took great courage too, as it is incredibly challenging and stressful to be with a dying child and their family. Ideally, the nurses were there to save lives, to make people better. It is understandable that because everyone loved him, they didn't want to let Arvind die. It is not surprising to learn that the staff found the experience emotionally draining.

Death is still a taboo subject and it is a challenge to engage in discussion with staff about how they feel, about their hopes and fears concerning the care of a child who is dying. On one hand they do want to talk and on another they find it almost too difficult and painful. Maybe on some level they deem it necessary to remain professional and competent and, therefore, worry that if they 'let go' and talk about how they feel, and the challenges they face, somehow they will break down and not be able to cope. In the process of wanting to do a good job there is perhaps a fear of 'getting it wrong', or losing control. Often staff fear saying the wrong thing or offending the people they are working with, and potentially find this even more difficult in situations such as when treatment is being withdrawn. Because of the overriding expectation that patients will be cured, even though they know that in reality some children will die, when death does occur they can feel that they have somehow failed. This is really difficult to cope with and, sadly, something very rarely acknowledged or voiced openly.

Important aspects of care

Emotions were running high and the family felt like they couldn't go on without Arvind. They were worried about each other and also about fulfilling Arvind's last wishes. Even so, Arvind's family appreciated all of the care and support they were offered in the hospital.

What the family valued most:

- being able to visit and stay with Arvind whenever they wanted

- staff being understanding and sensitive to their feelings and needs

- staff being honest and open

- a teacher who helped Arvind create a memory book, which the family can cherish for ever

- staff explaining what was happening and what was going to happen when Arvind died

- being given the opportunity to celebrate Christmas together with staff, family and friends and fulfil one of Arvind's final wishes

- the opportunity to give Arvind a bubble bath after he died, to dress him in his favourite t-shirt and to spend time with him before the funeral

- people showing emotion in front of them, as it showed they cared and were human

- staff respecting their wishes and actively listening

- staff going out of their way to pop in and just say hello.

Spiritual care is for everyone

Spiritual care is an important part of a child's wellbeing, just as physical and psychological support are. Potentially with any illness or trauma, and particularly with life-threatening illness, many spiritual questions might arise for the child and their family. 'What happens when we die?' 'Why me?' 'Is there life after death?' These questions can cause the child and their family great distress and anxiety, which can present as both physical and emotional pain. Some people would call this spiritual pain. Spiritual support is certainly not about giving easy answers; it is about actively listening and offering a contained, safe space for the questions to be voiced, which can be both powerful and empowering. Indeed, there are often no clear-cut answers and it is important to be honest about that. Because of this, being able to 'stay with' patients and their families in their struggles, questions and uncertainties takes great courage and commitment.

Listening carefully to the story of the child and the family is key to being able to offer the best possible spiritual care. The spiritual dimension is unique in each of us and we all express our spirituality in different ways. Spiritual care is about valuing and respecting who people are, whatever their culture, background, gender or sexuality. Spiritual care isn't about turning up with tick lists but about being there, in the ordinary and in the extraordinary, noticing both the spoken and the unspoken messages.

The danger of asking someone's religion and then ticking a box is that you never really find out what is important to them about their religion, or what they believe. It is important not to make assumptions about what people want and need, but instead allow people space to tell their story. Only by listening to the story of the child and family can the chaplain, teacher, nurse or doctor respond appropriately and sensitively.

Good communication is essential for all healthcare professionals: being clear about what is happening to the patient, being aware of the language we use and also checking out with the child and family what their understanding of the situation is. Families often have to face the unknown and uncertainty over what is happening to their child. Often, all the families want is to know that they are being heard and that their point of view is respected. They also want the staff working with them to be honest.

As a healthcare professional, whether it is as chaplain, teacher or nurse, part of our role often involves accompanying a patient and their family into the unknown: sometimes into scary places, where maybe there are no answers, all of which may increase anxiety and fear. We need to be able and willing to face the uncomfortable places as we walk alongside others. This can involve risk to oneself. Often working in such environments leads us to be acutely aware of our own lives and experiences, rekindling our own sense of loss, anxiety and fear. This may lead to the danger of wanting to run away from the pain and distress of others, as it may feel too much to bear. It is important to be aware of our own feelings and thoughts and, where possible, seek supervision and support. As Ewan Kelly says:

> finding ways for ourselves as carers to be able to sustain our humanity and ability to be vulnerable with others over time is crucial for our personal well-being and vocational fulfilment as much as it is for the quality of the care we provide. We need to find and maintain the balance between becoming swamped and overwhelmed by the wounds of others and distancing ourselves from them.[5]

Conclusion: in Shushma's words

My brother Arvind was rushed into his local hospital as he had Duchenne Muscular Dystrophy. After two weeks the doctor told us they could not save Arvind. We were told about the chaplain who worked in the hospital, but we were apprehensive at first as we were not very religious, but decided to let the chaplain come and visit. We were so glad that we did as we were introduced to Claire. She very quickly built up a bond and rapport with the whole family, so much so that we asked her to conduct Arvind's funeral. Claire listened as we grieved and supported us by respecting how we grieved. This was very important as many friends and professionals were telling us how we should grieve. She respected our wishes about not being that religious but still managed to support us and Arvind in the most difficult time in our lives. More importantly she built memories that will last with us forever. She made sure Arvind's final wishes took place like a Super Hero party and a Christmas party, where Claire lit candles, sang carols, decorated the chapel with Christmas decorations and got Santa to come in his sleigh. When Arvind passed away she came that day and supported us in the continuing days, so we could see Arvind. She made sure that when we went to see him he had his favourite duvet wrapped around him. We would have been lost without her.[6]

Notes

1   Kelly, E. (2012) *Personhood and Presence: Self as a Resource of Spiritual and Pastoral Care.* London: T&T Clark, p.100.

2   Allan, N. (1996) *Jesus' Christmas Party.* London: Red Fox.

3   Adapted from Galloway, K. (ed.) (1997) *The Pattern of our Days: Liturgies and Resources for Worship.* Glasgow: Wild Goose Publications, p.161.

4   Morley, J. (1998) *All Desires Known.* London: SPCK, p.112.

5   Kelly, E. (2012) *Personhood and Presence: Self as a Resource of Spiritual and Pastoral Care.* London: T&T Clark, p.109.

6   With special thanks to Shushma and all of the family for allowing me to share their stories and experiences.

9

A BUDDHIST MOTHER'S REFLECTIONS ON SPIRITUAL AND RELIGIOUS CARE

Kusumavarsa Hart

My experience of becoming a mother

After almost six years of trying for a child I became pregnant in January 2010. Having miscarried early on twice before, the first few weeks were filled with anxiety. At nine weeks pregnant the morning sickness became intolerable and an admission to hospital overnight revealed that I was pregnant with twins. I remember feeling excited and terrified at the same time. The journey through motherhood would be a challenging one and I would, in the weeks and months to come, rely on my faith as a Buddhist more than I could have imagined.

Prior to my pregnancy I was in the process of studying Buddhist psychology. My faith in Buddhism grew during my time as a student, and I had set upon the path of aspirant, or 'seeker', with a view to becoming a chaplain in the Amida Order, a Pureland Buddhist group based in the UK. Pureland Buddhism teaches a personal relationship with Amitaba Buddha who symbolizes mercy and wisdom. It also teaches a belief in the 'Pureland', which is an otherworldly place where liberation can take place.

By the time I was pregnant I felt I knew my path. I thought I had a deeper understanding of suffering and impermanence, two major Buddhist beliefs which teach us that suffering is realistic and happens to everyone, and that the roots of suffering are caused by greed, ignorance and destruction. Suffering can come from attachment to things that are not constant, that are in flux, including life itself – life is impermanence.

Childbirth and becoming a mother for me was not a joy, it was a horror story. There were small windows of beauty, but for most of the first 12 months of their little lives I was dragged to the lowest depths of my being and I felt pain in my heart so deep that I thought I might die. At 26 weeks and 4 days I had experienced some unusual back pain, had been sick during the night and was leaking some small amounts of fluid. I had not realized until it was too late that this meant there was something wrong. I was in the middle of teaching a workshop at the time and I decided I would try to get through the day and would call the hospital later to see if I should get checked out. The Amida Buddhist Order wear red at times of ceremony and when the community comes together. While it was not at the time a requirement for me to do so until after ordination, there were times I would wear red when I felt I needed to be close to Amida. This particular day was one of those days, and looking back I often wonder if there was a sense in me that I might need some extra support that day.

It was a beautiful, sticky hot Sunday, and I had been relaxed through most of the morning with no pain, refreshed from the meditations I had been teaching. At lunch I sat talking with my students. I stood up and, without warning, my waters broke, flooding the garden beneath my feet. Everyone sat in shock for a moment and I remember saying, 'I think my waters have broken but that can't be, it's too early.' The rest of the day was a ball of chaos as my husband Garry and I raced home in the car to get my hospital bag before heading to the Birmingham hospital where I had been due to give birth. I sat in the car on a wet towel that was soaking up the fluid that had held these little lives inside me and I felt overwhelmed with fear. I felt so helpless, so powerless, but I knew that staying calm was the most important thing that I could do. It was at that moment that my enlightenment began. I had two choices. I could let the primitive feelings of anger and anxiety kick in with full force, and live in pure ignorance in the hope that things would be OK, or I could offer myself up to Amida Buddha and put faith in an 'Other Power' and believe that all is as it should be. I had packed my *wagesha* and *mala beads*, two items I use in my practice, in my hospital bag ready.

Controlling terror through chanting

It became clear very early on after admission that I could not stay at the hospital I had planned to give birth in, and the closest with the required facilities was Sheffield. I tried to think of anyone I might know there and then there came the name 'Sundari'. We had met only a few times but as a minister with the Amida Order I wasn't afraid to ask her for help. I called the Buddhist House in Narborough where the Amida Order was gathered for an intensive few days of meetings. To hear Sundari's voice immediately put me at ease. 'I will meet you there. Garry can stay at our house,' she said. Her voice alone was a place of refuge and later her companionship and home also became a place of calm in an otherwise senseless and desperate time.

From my perspective as a Buddhist practitioner I was able to sit with the terror of my experience without becoming overwhelmed by it. I imagined the Amida Buddha and the *Bodhisattva* Quan Yin there, not far from me. And I hoped that everything would be all right – and by all right I mean as it should be. This meant whether the children lived or died I had to keep my faith that I would be supported by an 'Other Power' in this space of physical and mental suffering that I now found myself in. I knew that if they weren't going to make it, and the odds were seriously slim, then my practice was going to be so important to me and I couldn't think beyond that.

Different Buddhists will chant in different ways, and it's the feeling and intention behind the chant that matters. I chant *Oh mani padme hum* – a Quan Yin chant. Quan Yin is the *bodhisattva* of compassion and I would chant to her and imagine my two beautiful babies sitting on a lotus flower beside her, healthy and happy. I kept this visualization throughout their time in the neonatal unit. I felt for a long time that I was being held in a contained space, and this gave me a great sense of comfort and helped me to feel grounded in an otherwise terrifying ordeal. I never once lost the sense of an 'Other Power' beside me, and in my darkest hours I would say my faith endured with unwavering strength. When I am calling out 'Namo Amida Buddha' it means, 'This is all I am, this is all I have, I am calling out to you, Buddha.' You call out for help, for direction and to be held spiritually.

At 3.30am on Monday 28 June 2010 I was finally wheeled into an ambulance and driven to the other hospital in Sheffield. A nervous and rather anxious midwife sat beside me and her conversation that was designed to distract me only made me more anxious. I could see my blood pressure rising on the monitor. I said to her that I was going to do some mindfulness meditation and chanting, and I would let her know when I got a contraction. She looked a little puzzled but was happy to let me continue. My blood pressure began to normalize again and I felt relieved.

I tried to put to the back of my mind the fact that I had not felt one of my twins move for some time, praying all would be well. Having spent some time chanting to Quan Yin, I looked up to feel the gentle breeze from the window on my face. It felt cleansing, a welcome break from the intense heat of the daylight hours. It was the middle of the night and I was exhausted. I wondered how my body would cope with the next few hours. I felt a brief moment of anxiety rush in as I grasped a true sense of impermanence. I looked up to see in the reflection of the window a brilliant white full moon. I was captivated by its intensity. How had I missed it in the sky until now? I felt at that moment that Quan Yin was with me and that when the sunrise appeared Amida would be there to hold my heart as the day unfolded. When we finally arrived at the maternity unit the doors of the ambulance were flung open to the humid heat of the day once more. It was 5.30am and as anticipated the sunrise was beautiful, and if I never saw another again I would hold that one forever in my heart.

On Monday 20 June 2010 the twins were born by Caesarean section. Their fragile little bodies were rushed away without a sound. As I arrived in the recovery room two visions in red appeared within minutes – my *dharma* sisters Susthama and Sundari. They had left Narborough in the early hours to meet us, and those first few hours of support were so precious. In the days that followed the Amida Order sent two priests every day to see me, each taking time away from the Amida gathering to share in some of my suffering. They were all chanting for our children before morning service and I felt the power of their prayers within me.

Dharma brothers and sisters brought with them prayer cards and a statue of Quan Yin, and I used these priceless gifts to create a small shrine in the hospital room I was given. I named our children Ethan and Grace. The day after they were born we received life-changing news. We were ushered into a cosy room on the neonatal unit, where soft comfy sofas are designed to cushion the blow of bad news. My husband and I both chose to sit on the harder seats, numb at the news that our little boy had had a stroke at some point in the womb, and as a result he had brain damage. In that moment I felt my heart tear into a thousand pieces. Everything I thought I knew about life, every hope, every dream, every plan I thought I had written for my life was gone in an instant. Life would never be the same again. Right there was impermanence. Two weeks later we were faced with the news that our daughter might die from a serious infection. At home, 13 weeks later, our little boy stopped breathing. My husband breathed into his tiny body to keep him alive until paramedics came. Another month for Ethan in the children's intensive care unit fighting for life, while Grace was still fighting for hers on the neonatal unit. The list of infections and near-death moments could fill this whole book, but I wanted to give you a brief insight into our suffering. For a long time death seemed to be a whisper a way, and it took a lot of faith and hope to see that our children might get a chance at life.

My Buddhism

I have not always been a Buddhist; I was raised a Christian. I first picked up a book on Buddhism while at art college in 1999, and for the next decade found myself drawn to the path but never fully committed to the idea of having any religion at all. I went to the Buddhist House in 2007 and immediately loved the simpleness of the Pureland tradition. Pureland Buddhism originated in India and is popular today in China and Japan. It is accessible to all and focuses on *nembutsu*, or recitation, as well as meditation and the relationship with Amitabha (Amida) Buddha, a monk who became enlightened so is now a Buddha. I liked the idea of *bombu* nature – that we are all normal human beings, not yet enlightened. We all make mistakes, so if you are having a bad day you can remind yourself of that. The Amida Buddha is the embodiment of enlightenment, compassion and wisdom. The person who realizes him- or herself as being truly human, ignorant and full of passions attains Buddhahood by virtue of Amida Buddha. It is nice because it says you don't need to take the blame for things, due to our inherent human nature.

Community and chaplaincy support

For some of the time that we were in hospital my husband had needed to return home and without Sundari's support I would have felt extremely isolated. A Buddhist chaplain and an experienced Buddhist psychologist, Sundari had the ability to sit and listen and hold my words and feelings for me. She made sure I was well fed as the vegetarian options in hospitals aren't exactly the most nutritious for a vegetarian Buddhist mother who was trying to express milk for two babies! I remember one of the meals she brought was the most beautiful and nutritious lunch, a jacket potato with halloumi cheese and lots of salad leaves from her garden. It felt like a meal made with love; it was a simple gesture for her but to me it brought much needed nutrition and strength. It was also a reminder of the meals shared as a *sangha*, or community, with other Amida friends, a picture in my mind to draw strength from. However, she couldn't be there all the time and during our stays in hospital, no one ever asked us as a family if we needed a chaplain.

My medical notes would have indicated that I was a person of faith and yet even in our darkest hours no doctors or nurses ever asked us if we needed spiritual support. My own experience of being in hospital shaped my decision to train to be a chaplain. Although I was already on the aspirancy or seeker/student path, I had never really considered where my spiritual work might take me. It is only now looking back that I realize I needed to experience the journey I had with my own children in order to appreciate the spiritual needs of families, which are often very different from those of an adult staying in hospital. Because we now live in such a secular society I wonder if at times medical staff think that faith is only for the elderly and not the young? I also wonder if medical staff fully understand the role of a chaplain. Do they think that they are just there to give prayers for the sick and the dying? The role of the chaplain is much more than that.

Our darkest hour came two weeks after the twins were born when we were told that Grace might die. It was at this point I found myself picking up the phone once more and asking my friend and *dharma* sister Susthama Kim if she could come and bless the children. It was a very quiet, informal ceremony which we performed for both the twins. We chose a chant for each of them and my husband and I wrote a few short words for them both. We knew the future was uncertain for the twins but this simple ceremony that was truly heartfelt sealed the twins' connection with the *dharma*. For us as parents it helped us to let go of some of our fears. Giving all that you hold in your heart to the Buddha is a powerful part of the healing process at times like this.

After two bowel operations Grace slowly began to recover. Our daughter spent 14 months in hospital in total and we travelled between three different hospitals. In the months Grace spent in hospital my eventual encounters with both Christian and Buddhist chaplains were the most nourishing for me as a human being, a mother and as a person of faith. Visits from the Christian chaplain were always refreshing. She somehow used to magically appear when I was at my lowest. After months in hospital you become very institutionalized and often our conversations would turn to the world outside, to nature, to her hens and their egg-laying skills. The time with her was also the time when I could share my worst fears and my anger. She listened without judgement, helped me find my smile and we shared our common ground – the love of an 'Other Power' and the strength that can be gained from our faiths in these difficult times.

Space to chant and meditate

As a Buddhist finding a space to practise is often a challenge. None of the hospitals we experienced had a specific area for Buddhists, and the multifaith room often doesn't feel appropriate either. I tended to find myself migrating towards the Christian chapels, which are light and airy; the acoustics are perfect for practising the *nembutsu*, the ancient practice of chanting the Buddhist's name. If you find that you are resigned to the ward, unable to leave due to your child being too ill, then often there is no space at all in which you can practise, although there were times of emotional turmoil when I felt I had to walk up and down the ward mumbling the *nembutsu* while my daughter slept. In the process I hoped that the merit from my practice would help all the families on the ward and not just my daughter.

The ward was a godless place

When you spend months on a ward with your child, you see people come and go and you hear and see things that you wish you had not. When you are present on a particularly challenging day you wish that an 'Other Power' would touch the hearts of all the staff, family and the child. To allow your heart to be touched by the 'Other' known as God or Buddha is a transformational moment, when we can only hope that those who are suffering feel compassion and love enter their being. I remember I wrote on my blog after a particularly difficult day that 'the ward feels like a godless place'. This seems a harsh statement but the reality is that many patients and their families are helped on a medical level but receive very little support emotionally and spiritually. There are moments when sitting with a chaplain becomes a valuable support, a lifeline in the unfathomable landscape of your child's sickness and suffering. These are the times when you want someone to just come and sit and *be* with you, to allow you to say, 'I can't do this anymore.' I wanted someone to give us the opportunity to be afraid and to stop being strong for my daughter for just a minute, to let us be vulnerable in order to gain some strength.

View of suffering

I will always be so grateful for the specialist neonatal care we had access to, but I can't help thinking sometimes that this medical care is a double-edged sword. There are times when you think we play God with these small children, these little lives. Doctors make the decision to save these children and there is sometimes a price to pay for that, for both the child and the family. I can't think of many families I have met where the premature child is alive but free of complications because of the trauma they have gone through, as well as other issues unique to premature babies. It's difficult because life is precious, really precious, and you want to hold on to it, but at what cost? As a Buddhist you don't want anyone or anything to suffer, but you see your children go through horrendous suffering because of the nature of their early birth, and you can't do anything about it but pray. But what am I praying for? That it will hurt less? That they will forget it? Or that this won't linger in the rest of this life?

There were times when I felt that the doctors did not really understand the implication of procedures to a family of Buddhist faith, when our practice leads us daily to reflect on suffering and impermanence. At one time it was thought that because the premature baby's nervous system hasn't formed like a fully grown child, procedures could be done without anaesthetic. Even basic pain relief isn't used at times when you might think it would be.

The world of the premature baby is mostly a complex one from an ethical point of view, and in my opinion the premature baby is still regarded as an experiment. While science may say that their physical body doesn't feel pain, what is the psychological impact? Even the lack of acknowledgement of your child's name at times makes you feel that to the medical establishment your child is just another body, not a living, breathing beautiful human being who is fighting to survive. One day I couldn't take it any longer and I said to this one doctor, 'You never use her name, you never say, "Hello, Grace." This child is nearly 40 weeks old, and all you do is come in, stick a needle in her foot, and walk away. You never give her your name. Do you think she can't hear you?' He just said, 'I've never thought about that before.'

It must be horrific on a daily basis to look after these premature babies, but there must be a way to be more human and less blinkered towards the babies and the family. As a family you grieve the moments of childbirth that you will never have. I will never hold a full-term child of my own. My only memories are of my twins with tubes and monitors attached to their fragile bodies. These are our babies and even if you think as a medical professional that they do not suffer because they are not full term, we as parents carry their pain. How can I live with the pain and grief of suffering, and the anger? My whole world has been ripped apart and I've been left with two children with disabilities.

As a Buddhist I am grateful for the teachings on suffering. As a Buddhist there is no time to sit and say, 'Why me?' It is a time to say, 'Why *not* me?' Without my faith I think I would have broken down. Buddhism, including mindfulness-based work, talks about sitting with suffering. This is different from other faiths – they might say, have hope, pray to God and you will be helped. When you encounter great suffering it is painful, but it is also transformational. Life will never be the same but I can honestly say that I never really lived my life until the day my children were born. I thought I knew what pain and grief were. I thought I knew what suffering was but I did not. The last three years have shown me what real suffering is. No one wants to see their children in pain, hanging on to life, but in those fragile and precious moments I saw the power of the human spirit. There were so many times in both my children's lives when they could have died, and I strongly believe that they chose to live, and in that living they have taught me so much about life, love, death and faith.

Keeping my babies happy and safe

During our 14 months in hospital with my little girl, we constantly asked ourselves, 'How do we keep Grace's world happy and safe?' Routine becomes important. With Ethan at home I had no choice but to leave most of Grace's care to the nursing staff in hospital. There was no other choice; I did what I could to be the best mother and carer I could in the precious time we had. Our hospital visits included time spent chanting, reading, playing and going for walks as often as we could. As my Buddhist beliefs constantly encourage me to ask questions about ethics and suffering, I had some ethical concern around the food and medication Grace was being given. Where was the milk sourced from, was it powdered and did it come from a big brand with questionable ethics? The medication would have been tested on countless numbers of animals. I found myself having to weigh up the suffering as they saved her life. Maybe Grace will do something wonderful with her life that will balance this out from a karmic point of view.

I have been a vegetarian for the last 23 years and on becoming a Buddhist I also vowed not to eat meat or harm a sentient being. When the dietician decided that Grace could wean, the staff didn't ask me if I had any preferences, because they didn't realize my beliefs might affect this decision, so she was fed cottage pie. Staff knew I was Buddhist as I had a shaved head at the time and they had seen me chanting, but they didn't realize my beliefs extended to these practical decisions. When I found out, I went into meltdown – I was not prepared for this as all along we had believed she would not eat meat, at least in the short term. As the months and years have gone on and Grace continues to be predominately tube fed a formula milk, I have relaxed my attitude. Food gives us the gift of life, and to see Grace eat any food is a precious moment.

My children and the Buddha

From an early age Ethan has responded with great excitement when he sees a Buddha statue. At home I encourage the twins, who are now three, to clean the Buddha statues. Ethan likes to arrange them on a shelf in a particular way and he likes to leave small stones by an Amida Buddha that sits in the corner of the garden. At night before bed he often asks me to chant and he now joins in chanting *Namo Quan Shi Yin Bosat* – he is almost word perfect. It means 'I call out to the *bodhisattva* who listens with mercy to the sounds of the world.'

He connects on a deeper level with the Buddha and understands the love and compassion that comes with the *nembutsu*. Once I was upset after a very difficult day and he looked at me as tears came to my eyes and said, 'Mummy, remember the Buddha.' At the time he was only about two-and-a-half years old, and to me this was a powerful connection made in someone so young. He knew that I typically chanted at that time of night while they were getting changed for bed and must have realized the power of chanting for keeping me calm and happy.

Concluding thoughts

It is essential to find a way to engage with people in hospital and to tell them what chaplaincy is; that it's not about being forced into a belief but it's about support, emotional and spiritual. If the staff had a greater understanding of how a chaplain could help families then a greater connection could be made. It would be good to offer something to staff, such as Buddhist meditation, as part of staff education about religion. Buddhist chaplaincy can offer specific tools around mindfulness or meditation for staff through pre- or post-shift classes.

As I write this I know that another week-long trip to a hospital is imminent, this time for my son. I will no doubt pack my *wagesha, mala* beads and a small Buddha for the occasion. For any parent of a sick or disabled child, it is the threads of our faith (if you have one) that hold us together as we bravely hold our children through the path of adversity that they experience every day of their lives. As a Buddhist mother I know that impermanence can rush in at any moment. I try not to worry about the future; it is an unknown. I pray for stability, love and peace for the life we have right now, in this moment, and that is all that any of us can do.

10

ENGAGING HEALTH AND RELIGIOUS CARE TOGETHER

Paul Nash

So now you have read this book, what might be reasonable questions to ask and objectives to set to provide effective multifaith paediatric care?

- How can I take seriously and integrate the religious beliefs that might be important to families in my care, and how might those beliefs affect their care?

- How can this information be recorded and actioned?

- How can the asking for and implementation of this information be integrated into the patients' other care plans and records?

- What are the risks and benefits of doing this?

Sadly, there has been very little research into religious paediatric care, with most of the available material not differentiating between adults and children. In this chapter, we will share some of the tools and resources we are currently using and researching.

If we think about how healthcare happens, it has several common steps. When the patient presents their concerns and symptoms to you, in minimal terms the steps could be described as:

1. Diagnosis of the symptoms.

2. Organizing/planning further assessments and reviewing options.

3. Treatment/interventions: medical, psychological, etc.

4. Evaluation or assessment of treatments.

Religious care for children and their families in hospital should follow a similar robust pathway.

1. *Fact finding*: Asking for any religious affiliation.

2. *Assessment*: Identifying both the children's and families' specific needs.

3. *Intervention*: Facilitating, supporting and implementing articulated and identified needs.

4. *360 degree appraisal*: Assessing how effectively the needs have been meet.

Stages 2–4 may well be repeated on a regular basis as assessment needs to be ongoing.

Because of the wide-ranging contexts of the readers of this book, it is inappropriate and impossible to recommend one approach. For instance, the systems in the USA are on the whole far more developed in using these kinds of tools, so we do not want to teach anyone to 'suck eggs'. We also use and mean our words differently; religious and spiritual; multifaith and interfaith can mean different things according to context.

Paediatric context

As we said in Chapter 1, one of the distinctives of paediatric religious care is the involvement of the patient's family, because they are their guardians and some children are too sick or too young to express their own needs. This is no excuse for not engaging with the children, but a helpful assessment of one of the particularities of supporting sick, disabled and dying children and young people. Most of the tools mentioned in this chapter will be suitable for older patients and their parents. We describe two tools that we have particularly developed to engage children of any age.

What are we seeking to find out?

Do the child and/or the family have any religious:

- *Affiliation*: Would they self-identify themselves and follow a recognized religious belief and/or belong to a local religious community? (e.g. I am a Muslim, I am a Roman Catholic…)

- *Needs*: What do they believe would be affected by being in hospital or being ill? (e.g. Where can I go to pray? Is there food that conforms with my religious dietary laws? Are there any religious issues with the treatment I am being offered?)

Religious affiliation should be asked of all patients and families upon admittance. We know from our many years of experience that this is not always done because of several reasons. For example, staff do not ask because:

- they are too embarrassed or uncomfortable discussing faith

- they do not feel that it is appropriate to ask

- they do not feel they have the right language

- the admission was originally an emergency and some of the usual protocols were not followed.

There are many benefits of asking about their religious affiliation. For example, patients and families will know that their religion is important to the hospital. Also, the patients are more easily identified for visiting by the chaplaincy/spiritual care team.

Staff training, offered with sensitivity, can address some of the fears and ambivalence experienced when dealing with religious care.

If your unit or institution is seeking to enquire about religious affiliation as a part of history-taking or screening for religious needs, the most effective practice has been found to ask the questions using positive language such as:

'We have a very supportive chaplaincy team which includes members from your faith background. Would you like them to visit you and tell you about the facilities we have here?'

Offering patients and their families a leaflet which summarizes the religious and spiritual care offered can also be helpful.

Religious care pathways and care plans

The principle of this tool is to research the key aspects of care in each religious belief, design this into a pathway of questions for a member of staff to follow and then fill in the personalized care plan for that patient and/or family (see Appendix 3 for an example). At the time of writing, we are at the second stage of piloting and implementing these into our other pathways. In evaluation, staff have informed us that the questions are very helpful in giving them a language and a tool to offer care in areas in which they previously had very little knowledge.

The same five headings are used for all the types of pathway:

1. Communication

2. Personal care

3. Diet and food

4. Religious support/artefacts

5. Environment

We have written four different pathways to cover the four different stages of treatment, when the information needed may change:

1. Day to day

2. Palliative

3. End of life

4. Bereavement

Pathways have been written for six major world faiths (as in this book) but can be written for any faith.

The care plan uses the same five headings as the pathway, and is then adapted for individual patients. It invites the staff member to use questions around the five headings to find out what this particular family needs and how they would like to be supported in their religious care. Staff receive basic information and training in paediatric care for a particular faith and how to use the pathways and care plans.

Example: Islamic palliative care pathway

1. Communication

    -   Interpreter

    -   Decision-making

2. Personal care

    -   Same-gender care

    -   Personal hygiene

-   Clothing and modesty

3. Diet and food

    -   Medication and cures

4. Religious support/artefacts

    -   Visit from a religious leader

    -   Religious and spiritual needs

    -   Visitors

5. Environment

    -   Conducive environment

    -   Visual space

    -   Care in the community

The example in Appendix 3 is for Islamic palliative care and the headings reflect the particular needs of this faith group at the palliative stage in treatment.

Benefits of pathways

-   They help staff to take a patient's religious identity and needs seriously.

-   They give staff the confidence to know they have some of the basic information they need to have an informed conversation with a patient's family.

-   The care plans are personalized for every family, and therefore no assumptions are made.

-   Different pathways can be followed as the condition of the child changes, so that other aspects can be taken into account.

We have designed these so far for the six faiths mentioned in this book for daily, palliative, end-of-life and bereavement care. At BCH, we also offer training sessions including simulation with dolls and virtual rooms with additional information booklets for staff.[1]

Religious and spiritual assessment and interventions with children and young people

Another model we have developed at BCH, which takes into account the age and developmental level of children and young people, is a range of activities which give children the opportunity to explore spiritual and, as appropriate, religious needs. We have found this more narrative approach to be helpful in eliciting such information as how they are feeling and what is important to them.[2]

Beads bracelet

An example of this is our beads bracelet, which we often use as an initial activity with a new child or young person. We take along a box of different coloured beads and have a card which goes with each one where each coloured bead represents a different aspect of spiritual care, one of which is to be loved by God. When the child has made the bracelet, they are invited to tell the staff member about it. In some cases the child uses overtly religious language to describe the beads, in other cases just spiritual, but some take the opportunity to identify the qualities they don't have but need or want. These worksheets can be easily modified to change the name of God to make them more accessible to other faiths. See Appendix 4 for one version of this activity.

Hear my prayer postcard

Using a picture of large satellite dishes on a clifftop (which is not religious-specific and ideally attractive to both genders) and the words, 'There's always someone listening…hear my prayer,' children are invited to write their own prayer on the reverse side of the postcard. They may then pray their prayer, invite a chaplain to pray it or ask the staff member they are working with to give it to a chaplain or put it in chapel so someone else prays their prayer. An actual example of such a prayer can be found in Appendix 4.

Family activities and conversations

We have also designed activities to be done by whole families to give the opportunity to explore religious and spiritual needs. What these activities do is give an easy way into having a conversation about what is important to the whole family and to different members of the family. These have given us the opportunities for families to share religious beliefs, how they impact and how they view the child's illness.[3]

Other religious history-taking, screening and assessment of religious needs tools

There are several tools available and these may seek to achieve initial screening of a patient's religious history; identify what has helped in the past; or seek to assess their needs now in the light of their medical condition and their faith beliefs; and identify how they can now be supported.

Religious and spiritual screening and history-taking is when initial questions are asked by a healthcare professional including a chaplain, although chaplains are more likely to do a spiritual assessment.[4] These are some of the popular tools:

The HOPE questions

H: What are the patient's sources of hope, meaning, comfort, strength, peace, love and connection?

O: What role does organized religion have for the patient?

P: What is the patient's personal spirituality and what practices does this include?

E: What are the effects of the patient's beliefs/spirituality on their medical care and end-of-life decisions?[5]

FICA: taking a spiritual history

The acronym FICA can help structure questions in taking a spiritual history by healthcare professionals.[6]

F: Faith and belief

'Do you consider yourself spiritual or religious?' or 'Do you have spiritual beliefs that help you cope with stress?' If the patient responds 'No', the physician might ask, 'What gives your life meaning?' Sometimes patients respond with answers such as family, career or nature.

I: Importance

'What importance does your faith or belief have in your life? Have your beliefs influenced how you take care of yourself in this illness? What role do your beliefs play in regaining your health?'

C: Community

'Are you part of a spiritual or religious community? Is this of support to you and how? Is there a group of people you really love or who are important to you?' Communities such as churches, temples and mosques, or a group of like-minded friends can serve as strong support systems for some patients.

A: Address in care

'How would you like me, your healthcare provider, to address these issues in your healthcare?'

Brief RCOPE

This is a short measure of religious coping in relation to major life stressors[7] and has been quite widely tested and validated. It is more overtly religious than some of the other tools. Participants are asked about both positive and negative elements of religious coping, identifying if they have done them not at all, somewhat, quite a bit or a great deal, for example.

Positive religious coping subscale items

1. Looked for a stronger connection with God.

2. Sought God's love and care.

3. Sought help from God in letting go of my anger.

4. Tried to put my plans into action together with God.

5. Tried to see how God might be trying to strengthen me in this situation.

6. Asked forgiveness for my sins.

7. Focused on religion to stop worrying about my problems.

Negative religious coping subscale items

1. Wondered whether God had abandoned me.

2. Felt punished by God for my lack of devotion.

3. Wondered what I did for God to punish me.

4. Questioned God's love for me.

5. Wondered whether my church had abandoned me.

6. Decided the devil made this happen.

7. Questioned the power of God.

IDENTIYING SPIRITUAL DISTRESS – A CHAPLAIN'S EXPERIENCE

I look for spiritual suffering in five areas: Love, Faith, Hope, Virtue and Beauty. Other names for these categories could be Connection, Worldview, Meaning/Purpose, Integrity/Ethics, Renewal. If a child's family relationships are in disarray, spiritual intervention is indicated as these are a large part of one's spiritual life. If faith questions loom large this is also an indication of spiritual suffering. Hope, itself powered by meaning and purpose, powers our spiritual resources of healing and reintegration. Virtue is a set of spiritual characteristics that aid in working with others to regain health. And our spiritual needs for beauty and humor and renewal are known well to occupational therapists and child life specialists; chaplains also do well to remember the 'imago dei' of our Creator. These five categories of spiritual need guide me as I travel alongside those in our hospital. (Rev Mark Bartel, Orlando, Florida)

Using tools

The objective of these tools is to ensure that the patient and/or family is asked these questions and that the relevant answers are recorded and taken into account in their care. The goals of these tools all have a place in our health and palliative care. Unfortunately, there is almost no research or evidence of what works well in paediatrics and hospices, for children, young people and their families. Our suggestion is you try out the range of approaches we describe here.

Whose role is this work?

With so much overlap between tasks and the diversity of roles within our institutions, this is an almost impossible question to ask, but an important one nevertheless. I like this apocryphal story:

> There was an important job to be done and Everybody was sure that Somebody would do it. Anybody could have done it, but Nobody did it. Somebody got angry about that because it was Everybody's job. Everybody thought that Anybody could do it, but Nobody realized that Everybody wouldn't do it. It ended up that Everybody blamed Somebody when Nobody did what Anybody could have done.

The following offers a guide only:

- *Religious affiliation*: hospital administrators upon admission
- *Religious referrals, history and screening*: nurses and healthcare support staff
- *Religious assessment*: chaplains and other spiritual care staff
- *Religious interventions*: chaplains, local religious leaders, other staff as appropriate.

All the information needs to be recorded and referrals made as necessary. However, what is most important is not what things are called but that they get done. It is important that religious needs are taken seriously and integrated into care plans or pathways, and staff are aware of the religious beliefs that are important to families and how this might affect their care. This information should be recorded and actioned, assessments should be ongoing, and the asking and implementation of this information should be integrated into the patient's other care plans and records. Taking the religious needs of the patients and their families seriously serves to enhance patient care and often contributes positively to patient satisfaction.

Notes

1   Further information on this and details of training offered can be obtained from Red Balloon Resources. Email: rbr@bch.nhs.uk.

2   This is affirmed by Thayer, P and Nee, R. (2009) in 'Spiritual Care of Children and Parents.' In A. Armstrong-Dailey and S. Zarbock (eds) *Hospice Care for Children* (3rd edn). Oxford University Press, pp.219–239. They identify some of the pertinent issues in spiritual care in this setting.

3   See Nash, P., Darby, K. and Nash, S. (2015) *Spiritual Care for Sick Children and Young People*. London: Jessica Kingsley Publishers for a comprehensive introduction to the topic and lots of examples of such activities, some of which are available to buy. Email: rbr@bch.nhs.uk.

4   A useful overview of some of the most popular ones is to be found in Christina Puchalski (2010) 'The Spiritual History: An Essential Element of Patient-Centred Care.' In McSherry, W. and Ross, L. (eds) *Spiritual Assessment in Healthcare Practice*. Keswick: M&K Publishing. The summaries presented here are based on those found in this book.

5   See Anandjarah, G. and Hight, E. (2001) 'Spirituality and medical practice using the HOPE questions as a practical tool for spiritual assessment.' *American Family Physician 63*, 1, 81–89 for a full overview.

6   See Puchalski, C. and Romer, A.L. (2000) 'Taking a spiritual history allows clinicians to understand patients more fully.' *Journal of Palliative Medicine 3*, 1, 129–137 for a more detailed explanation.

7   See Pargament, K., Feuille, M. and Burdzy, D. (2011) 'The Brief RCOPE: Current psychometric status of a short measure of religious coping.' *Religions 2*, 51–76 for an overview.

CONCLUSION

Paul Nash

While this book seeks to introduce key beliefs from six world faiths relating to sick and dying children and their families, faith is diverse and the way individuals practise it may differ from what we have written. What is therefore important is to absorb and adopt general principles which take religious faith seriously when seeking to engage and support children and their families in their healthcare.

A CHAPLAIN'S EXPERIENCE

It is important to remember the role differentiation between a hospital chaplain and the leaders of one's chosen religious tradition. Clergy have an authority as representatives of the tradition chosen. They will have a different relationship altogether, as they will most likely be seen as the authority in what to do and believe. The hospital chaplain, on the other hand, was not chosen by the patient or family. Rather, the chaplain comes with the hospital and has the role of accompanying the patient and family through the recovery process or death process. We may be seen as suspect by some traditions, while others may see chaplains as safer to speak to about their doubts or questions. Again, it is up to the individual to let us know what they need. (Rev Mark Bartel, Orlando, Florida)

In any such book there has to be some parameters for identifying which faiths to cover and with the limitations of space we have covered the six faiths with the highest populations in the UK at the time of writing. We are sure a similar resource for other world faiths and cultural groups would be a helpful contribution to facilitating more effective support of our patients and their families.

The 4Rs of multifaith care

Relationships

These are key in assessing and offering religious care in health and hospice care. Building trust and understanding are essential. This can be done even at the beginning when you do not understand anything about your patient's beliefs, but by asking, offering and listening, staff are able to engage with what might be very important to patients and affect their condition and wellbeing.

Resources

We can work towards ensuring we have bespoke resources to support and educate children, families and healthcare staff in religious and spiritual care. These need to take seriously the development levels of children and young people and how these might be impacted by their condition, and engagement with their faith. Bereavement resources need to be appropriate and reflect religious and spiritual beliefs where possible. Most resources for adults are not fit for purpose in a paediatric setting and we need to ensure that what we offer is a comfort to them.

Rituals

Rituals are wonderful ways in which we seek to express our beliefs, with and without words. In healthcare, we need to find creative ways to facilitate religious rituals while children are bed-bound, on machines or are semi-mobile. We also consider how all the family (using that term in the widest sense) can be involved in rituals at significant times such as rites of passage and end of life.

Research

We need to commit ourselves towards evidence-based best practice in our multifaith daily, palliative, end of life and bereavement care. Much of our intuition and instinct is based upon a wealth of experience and knowledge, but for this type of care to be taken seriously within healthcare, we need to be able to evidence what works and what children, families and staff prefer and find is the most effective.

We hope this book makes a contribution towards developing knowledge, skills and attitudes in these areas.

Core principles

In conclusion, our core principles for best practice in paediatric multifaith care are:

1. Ask, never assume.

2. Act with compassion, with a non-judgemental attitude and personal integrity.

3. Have religious affiliation and assessment as an acknowledged integrated multidisciplinary system in your unit and institution. Ensure your systems and staff can record the patients' and families' religious affiliation, assessments and referrals.

4. Develop these tools for both patients of all ages and their families.

5. Be observant: what do you see around the room that might indicate religious belief might be important to this family?

6. Remind yourself there is diversity within diversity; no one Buddhist, Christian, Hindu, Jew, Muslim, and Sikh is exactly the same as another. Patients may also have different beliefs to those of their family and there may be different faiths within a family.

7. Be mindful of the overlap between religious, spiritual and cultural needs and care.

8. Seek to integrate continuous religious and health/palliative assessment and care.

9. Have regular religious and cultural celebrations.

10. Offer and refer on to religious care chaplains. Don't just wait for end of life.

11. Apologize when you get it wrong.

12. When training in the area of multifaith care use a SAKE framework; exploring Skills, Attitudes, Knowledge and Ethics. Have reference material available.

13. Be both gentle and mindful with yourself, you will never know it all, but seek to become more consciously competent and literate in multifaith care. Also be aware of how our own bias and beliefs could affect care.

14. Celebrate our common humanity.

Our experience and research suggests that we will use different tools and resources for families and children. Whatever tools we use for multifaith care assessment and planning, and implementing interventions, it is important that we move towards a robust, universal system that is understood by staff, families and children.

Let's be mindful that cross cultural/religious conversations and interactions can be confusing. Levels of global mobility suggest that we will be encountering new ways of practising particular faiths and fresh perspectives on multiculturalism. Let's commit ourselves that the only PC we are interested in fulfilling is patient-centred care – being respectful of others and treating others how we would like to be treated.

As we said in the Introduction, even as precise as we have sought to be in this book, we are not imagining we are covering the spectrum of all the different traditions within each of these world faiths. We hope to have made a contribution to taking children and young people as patients of faith seriously, and not just treating them like 'little adults'.

PALLIATIVE, END-OF-LIFE AND BEREAVEMENT ISSUES IN THE RELIGIOUS CARE OF CHILDREN

The following table contains broad guidelines only and it is vital to ask each family what their preferences are – *ask, don't assume.*

Copyright © Paul Nash (paul.nash@bch.nhs.uk), Chaplaincy, Birmingham Children's Hospital, March 2014

Issues	Buddhism	Christianity	Hinduism
Care of the dying and end of life	May not wish to have sedatives. Family may wish to wash the body. Provide a place and space of peace and quiet. Some families may wish for the body not to be touched for as long a possible after the death (time for the mind to leave the body).	Offer a Baptism or blessing for the child if this has not happened.	Any jewellery and sacred threads should not be removed. Close eyes and straighten body. Family may ask for the dying patient to be placed on the floor. Family may wish to wash the body and wrap it in a white cloth. Holy water may be applied to the lips.
Visit from the religious leader	Call a faith representative to facilitate peace and quiet for meditation.	Roman Catholics and some members of the Church of England require a priest for last rites, blessing and/or baptism.	A priest may be required, reading from holy books.
Organ donation	No religious preference as norm.	No religious preference as norm.	No main issues.
Post-mortem	No religious preference as norm.	No religious preference as norm.	No religious preference as norm.

Funeral	Cremation is preferred but will depend on tradition.	No general preference for burial or cremation.	Funeral take places as soon as possible after death. Children may be buried; adults are cremated. Gift of a toy in the coffin for the child to play with while they are in heaven awaiting rebirth. Photo and candle/religious symbol at home up for 12 days after funeral.
Beliefs about suffering	Suffering is universal and is eased by not being selfish.	Varied attitudes. Can be fatalistic or angry with God.	Varied attitudes.
Belief about the afterlife	Believe in rebirth.	Believe in life after death in heaven or hell. Infants assured of heaven in most traditions.	Believe in rebirth. Children enter heaven first.
Gender	Adapt to local culture.	No main differences.	Women wear *shari* at end of life. Only close female relatives at crematorium. Gender-to-gender greeting at home, using holy name of God.

Issues	Judaism	Islam	Sikhism
Care of the dying and end of life	May wish to hear Psalm 23 read and the *Shema*. The body should be handled as little as possible. After death, close eyes. Clothing is to remain and body covered with sheet. Hygienic washing can be completed by staff but religious washing will take place separately. Family may wish to wash body. Most traditions may wish for same gender contact only in preparing the body. Most traditions may wish for the child not to be left alone. Separate undertakers.	May wish for reading before death. Eyes and mouth closed, body straightened, head turned to the right and body covered with clean sheet. May wish to pray towards Makkah in Saudi Arabia. Privacy for family to grieve. Any sacred jewellery should not be removed. Washing has to be in accordance with Islamic faith. Families may wish to take the child home with them. Separate undertakers.	The 5Ks should not be removed. Family will read the holy books; there are no priests. Music or prayers may be played. Close eyes and straighten body. Family may wish to wash and dress the body. If the boy has been baptised as a Sikh, he will wear a turban. Young boys who have not been baptised may wear a head covering.
Visit from the religious leader	Offer a visit from a rabbi, but readings are normally led by the family.	Offer a visit from an *imam*, but prayers are normally led by the family.	Offer a visit from a priest or chaplain, but readings can be led by the family.
Organ donation	Varied attitudes; referral to rabbi.	Varied attitudes (allowed by majority).	Varied attitudes, generally OK.

Post-mortem	Varied attitudes; some families will be very much against it; referral to rabbi.	Not keen.	No main issues.
Funeral	Funeral takes place as soon as possible after death, within 24 hours. A 'watcher' sits with the body within some traditions. May prefer burial in separate cemetery. Mourners do not leave the house. Mourning for a child is 30 days.	Funeral takes place as soon as possible after death, within 24 hours. Always buried. Funeral prayer will be led by the *imam*. Believe in paradise or hell (young children assured of paradise and interceding for parents).	Always cremated, although babies without teeth may be buried. Mourners sometimes wear white. Ashes poured into flowing water.
Beliefs about suffering	Varied attitudes.	Death is seen as the will of God. Lifespan of every individual was allocated at the beginning of time. *Subr* (patience) is highly encouraged.	Varied attitudes.
Belief about the afterlife	Believe in life after death in heaven or hell. Infants assured of heaven in most traditions.	Believe in life after death in heaven or hell. Infants assured of heaven and pray for family.	Believe in rebirth.

Issues	Judaism	Islam	Sikhism
Gender	The Orthodox tradition will prefer same-gender care, touch, etc. Some traditions do not have women participating in mourning (Kaddish) prayer.	Segregation at funeral.	Eldest son represents family. Will sit separately at funeral.

KEY FESTIVALS

There are two lists, one of festivals which fall on a fixed date each year and the other where the date changes. This is a UK-focused list, based on the Western calendar; there may be other festivals and dates that are significant for families to celebrate depending on their religious and cultural practices.[1]

Celebration	Religious/cultural	Date
New Year's Day	Cultural	1 January
Birthday of Guru Gobind Singh	Sikh	5 January
Epiphany	Christian	6 January
Makar Sankrant	Hindu	14 January
St Valentine's Day	Cultural	14 February
St David's Day	Cultural – Wales	1 March
St Patrick's Day	Cultural – Ireland	17 March
Mahasivratri	Hindu	17 March
Birthday of Guru Nanak	Sikh	14 April
Vaisakhi	Sikh	15 April
St George's Day	Cultural – England	23 April
Lailat-ul-Barat	Muslim	2 June
Martyrdom of Guru Argen Dev ji	Sikh	16 June
Summer Solstice	Pagan	21 June
Halloween	Cultural	31 October
All Saints Day	Christian	1 November
Martyrdom of Guru Tegh Banabur	Sikh	24 November
St Andrew's Day	Cultural – Scotland	30 November
Christmas Day	Christian	25 December

Festivals with changing dates	Religious/cultural
Mawlid-un-Nabi	Muslim
Chinese New Year	Chinese
Shrove Tuesday/Mardi Gras	Cultural
Ash Wednesday	Christian
Holi	Hindu
Mothering Sunday	Christian
Good Friday	Christian
Passover	Judaism
Easter Sunday	Christian
Shri Rama Navami	Hindu
Yom Hashoah	Judaism
Shavuot	Judaism
Pentecost	Christian
Ascension Day	Christian
Ramadan	Muslim
Dharma day	Buddhist
Eid al Fitr (end of Ramadan)	Muslim
Raksha Bandhan	Hindu
Janamashtami	Hindu
Rosh Hashanah	Judaism
Hajj	Muslim
Eid-ul-Adha	Muslim
Yom Kippur	Judaism
Sukkot/Harvest	Judaism, Christianity
Navarati	Hindu
Deepavali (Diwali)	Hindu, Sikh, Jain
Al Hijira	Muslim
Birthday of Guru Nanak	Sikh
Advent Sunday	Christian
Hanukkah	Judaism

Note

1   The Interfaith Calendar website has a more comprehensive list of festivals
and can be used to check dates. Available at: www.interfaithcalendar.org

PALLIATIVE CARE PATHWAY

Islamic Faith Example

The following page shows an example palliative care pathway for a Muslim child and family.

Communication

Interpreter

If needed, use professional interpreters, not family members, where possible.

Decision-making

There may be a hierarchy in the family. Identify main decision-makers and key family members. Decisions are often made after consultation with the family rather than autonomously; allow time for this. Be aware of the mother's wishes, which may not in some cases hold priority in the process. Family may not wish child to know the decision.

Personal care

Same-gender care

Where possible for children over 10. Children reach adulthood at puberty of 15 years male, 9 years female. Care may be provided by opposite gender, if same-gender care not available.

Personal hygiene

Running water is required after the use of the toilet and for bathing. Nails are cut and pubic hair is removed. Blood, urine or faeces on body or clothing will render them impure. Ablution required for acts of worship. Full ritual bath required for end of menstruation or emission of sexual fluid. Alcohol and pig products should also be avoided.

Clothing and modesty

Males require covering from the navel to the knee and females the whole body except hands, feet and face, but some may include these also. Provide appropriate clothing and privacy, particularly for children over the age of 10. Segregated bed space is preferable.

Diet and food

Diet and food

Muslims require *halal* (permissible) food; this will include all vegetables and meat slaughtered in a *halal* method. All pig, alcohol and blood products and derivatives will be *haram* (impermissible). Touching of *halal* with any *haram* will make it impermissible. Allow food from home if possible. Certain food may be considered to help or hinder healing. Breast-feeding is of religious merit.

Medication and cures

Medication needs to be *halal*, however any product can be used if *halal* alternative is not available. Cures can be spiritual, such as verses of the Quran, supplications, holy water and charity.

Religious support/artefacts

Visit from religious leader

Not a requirement; family may make a request for an imam or Muslim chaplain. Extended family may need to know.

Religious and spiritual needs

Quran being recited around the bed; the use of prayer beads; display of holy scriptures, holy water; patient wearing amulets, giving of charity; family's need for prayer and purification. Provide prayer and ablution facilities for family. Quran treated with great respect. Muslims do not place it near feet, turn their backs or put anything on top of it. Do not remove amulets or holy scripture without permission.

Visitors

It is a religious duty to visit the sick, end-of-life visitors may increase – facilitate where possible. Death and dying is a communal event. Extended family may wish to be involved in care.

Environment

Conducive environment/visual space

No representation of humans or animals. No images of eyes. Space for visitors and readings. Some children may not be comfortable drawing images or having dolls and lifelike toys.

Care in the community

Considered a great virtue to look after the sick; extended family may be involved in the care. For home visits you may need to remove shoes. There may be dedicated prayer areas, please ask; females may not be comfortable being alone with a male member of staff.

EXAMPLES OF SPIRITUAL CARE ACTIVITIES

Making a bead bracelet for spiritual care

- Invite the child or young person to make a bead bracelet.

- Show them the beads in the box and 'explore' them.

- As appropriate, talk about colours, shapes, textures (the questions asked and the approach needs to be adapted to the age, gender and nature of illness of the child/young person).

- Talk about other pieces of jewellery the child/young person has.

- Who were they given by?

- Are they special or precious? If so, why?

- What does wearing their chosen jewellery express about themselves?

- Introduce the card which ascribes different feelings to different coloured beads and use it to begin to explore feelings about being in hospital (or contextualize as appropriate to faith, context, etc.).

- What is good about it? What makes them smile while in hospital?

- What is more difficult about being in hospital? What do they miss while away from home?

- With older children and young people use the colours and related ideas on the card as beads are selected (they could be placed in a 'sick bowl' until ready for threading). Take time to talk through each feeling, strength or quality. Discuss why and how each is important and how they 'see' it in practice.

- Once the bracelet is made, discuss the questions on the card as you encourage the child/young person to think about what they already have, what they are able to offer others and how they might get or grow the things they don't yet have…

Younger children

- With younger children beads can be chosen in other ways. For example, selecting beads that represent different things and people who are important to the child. Exploring 'why' the people and things they choose are important might be very revealing and lead into an opportunity to discuss ideas such as 'happiness', 'strength', 'belonging'…

- With children under five to six years old just listing the people that are important and knowing they are loved and safe with them will probably be enough.

Hear my prayer postcard

This is a prayer written by a seriously injured young woman in response to our card which has on the front, 'There's always someone listening…hear my prayer.' It was a religious prayer focusing on others rather than herself, despite her multiple needs at the time of writing. It illustrates the importance of allowing people to express their religious needs and identity which may include gratitude and a focus outside of themselves.

> Thank you Lord for this day that you gave me this day and thank you for all the children that are laid now in this hospital today. Make them better…also those going through worse, and for those who's getting out. Thank you Lord for everything you did for them. Make them to thank you. Then show them that you exist. Show them that you are there for them, that you're their Father. Thank you for everything that you did from when I come in till the last day I go away. Thank you, very, very much. Amen.

LIST OF RED BALLOON RESOURCES AND CONTACT DETAILS

Islamic resources

Leaflet for parents: *Your Child is in Hospital*

Booklet for staff: *Caring for the Muslim Child and their Family in Hospital* (32 pages)

Support for Muslim families who have been told their child is no longer curable: bag of activity sheets and cards for children, young people and families in hospital

Book for bereaved children: *We Will Meet Again in Jannah* (paperback gift book)

Book for bereaved parents: *A Gift for the Bereaved Parent* (hardback gift book)

Condolence card and anniversary of bereavement card

Sikh resources

Sikh Prayers for the Loss of a Child (paperback gift book)

Sikh Prayers for an Ill Child (hardback gift book)

Virtual training rooms (Moodle): for daily, end-of-life and bereavement care

Held in Hope series: story books for Christian children (for 3–7-year-olds): *Maya Goes to Hospital; Josh Stays in Hospital; Sam and his Special Book* (in life-limited care); *Jesus still Loves Joe* (bereavement care) £5.99 each

For further details

Rev Paul Nash

Chaplaincy

Birmingham Children's Hospital NHSFT

Steelhouse Lane

Birmingham

B4 6NH

0121 333 8526

rbr@bch.nhs.uk

ABOUT THE AUTHORS

Paul Nash has worked at Birmingham Children's Hospital since 2002 and has been Chaplaincy Team Leader (Senior Chaplain) since 2004. He is Director of Red Balloon Resources, for paediatric daily, palliative, end-of-life and bereavement care for children, families and staff and the Co-founder and Co-convenor of the Paediatric Chaplaincy Network for Great Britain and Ireland. Paul is perceived to be one of the leading thinkers in the field of paediatric chaplaincy. He is the academic lead on children's and young people's chaplaincy modules with Staffordshire and Gloucestershire Universities.

Madeleine Parkes is a spiritual care advisor and researcher with Birmingham and Solihull Mental Health NHS Foundation Trust and Birmingham Children's Hospital NHS Foundation Trust. She has worked as an autism therapist and volunteers with the Samaritans. She is continuing her counselling training with accreditation from the UK Council for Psychotherapists and has a keen interest in the role that spirituality and religion can play in health and wellbeing, particularly in mental health.

Zamir Hussain is a Muslim chaplain at Birmingham Children's Hospital and has pioneered resources in Islamic health care. She has published several books for bereaved Muslim parents and siblings. She has also developed the first UK blended learning resource, including care plans and pathways for Islamic daily, palliative, end-of-life and bereavement care for paediatric staff. Zamir has worked as a Muslim chaplain for both the Heart of England NHS Trust and Birmingham Children's Hospital for over five years.

THE CONTRIBUTORS

Mark Bartel is Chaplain Manager, Spiritual Care, Arnold Palmer Medical Center, Orlando, Florida, USA.

Thomas Begley is Lay Roman Catholic Chaplain to Laura Lynn Children's Hospice, Ireland.

Rakesh Bhatt is a Hindu Chaplain to Paediatric, Acute and Mental Health NHS Trusts, UK.

Rev Claire Carson is an Anglican Priest and Hospital Chaplain at St George's University Hospitals NHS Foundation Trust in London, UK.

Rev Kathryn Darby is Methodist Chaplain to Birmingham Children's Hospital, UK.

Kusumavarsa Hart is a therapist and writer based in the West Midlands, UK.

Rabbi Naomi Kalish is Coordinator of Pastoral Care & Education at the NYP Morgan Stanley Children's Hospital (New York, USA) and President of the National Association of Jewish Chaplains (NAJC).

Kelsang Leksang is a resident teacher at the Kadampa Meditation Centre, Birmingham, and Buddhist Chaplain to Birmingham Children's Hospital, UK.

Keith Munnings is a member of the Buddhist Healthcare Chaplaincy Group, UK.

Rabbi Meir Salasnik is Rabbi of Bushey and District United Synagogue, UK.

Satish K. Sharma is General Secretary of the National Council of Hindu Temples, UK.

Parkash Sohal offers Sikh chaplaincy services to Paediatric and Acute NHS services in the West Midlands, UK.

Dr Jaswant Singh Sohal is a retired dentist and offers advice about Sikh faith and practices, UK.

Surinder Sidhu works at Birmingham Children's Hospital, UK.

Yve White-Smith is a Palliative and End of Life Care Chaplain in the UK.

INDEX